DENTISTS AT WAR

12 WHO WENT BEYOND
THE CALL OF DUTY

Norman Wahl, DDS, MS, MA

authorHOUSE®

AuthorHouse™
1663 Liberty Drive
Bloomington, IN 47403
www.authorhouse.com
Phone: 1 (800) 839-8640

Published by AuthorHouse 06/11/2020

ISBN: 978-1-7283-6007-2 (sc)
ISBN: 978-1-7283-6006-5 (e)

Library of Congress Control Number: 2020907486

Print information available on the last page.

CONTENTS

FOREWORD

It has been said that life's meaning comes from three things: the love we can give, the work we can offer in times of crisis, and our ability to display courage in the face of suffering. The menace may be subhuman or superhuman, but we all have the option of asserting our own dignity even until the end. Such has been the challenge confronting Norm Wahl as he explored the lives of 12 dentists who served their country in times of peril. I urge you to read Norm's story of these hitherto unknown brave individuals whose timely service allows us to now live the healthy and productive lives we so cherish. Yes, they all happen to be dentists, but that distinction alone will serve to hold your attention when their common values of life were challenged by the unbelievable pressures that come with war.

Believe it or not, military dentistry was a necessity even before we had dentists, that is, during the American Revolution. But it was during the Civil War and again in World War I that dentistry had a major impact in saving lives. During World War II, dental officers were finally given a degree of status and often served as medical officers as well as dental officers. The wars in Korea and Viet Nam involved much larger engagement by dentistry as its members became fully involved from start to finish.

But who are the dentists who achieved the highest degree of recognition in Norm's account of history and for what reasons were they selected? More specifically, what makes an ordinarily peace-loving dentist, when confronted with the circumstances of war, rise to the occasion and perform acts of heroism? The answers are exemplified by these 12 dental officers, all of whom, in order to qualify for selection, needed three attributes: (1) They had a DDS or DMD, (2) They were members of the armed forces, and (3) Their feats were performed during time of war (WWI or WWII). In keeping with the historical nature of this account, the selectees are grouped by wars. Three carried out their exploits during WWI, one served in both world wars, and the other eight were involved in WWII. Of these eight, six were POWs; two were not. Of the six POWs, three were American, two were Scottish, and one was Dutch-American. They were

Weedon E. Osborne
Alexander G. Lyle
Varaztad H. Kazanjian
Bernard C. Freyberg
Jack H. Taylor
Coenraad F.A. Moorrees
Albert N. Brown
Roy L. Bodine Jr
Julius Morris Green
David Arkush
Benjamin Lewis Salomon
Robert E. Moyers

Perhaps the selectee who rates my greatest personal admiration is Robert Edison Moyers, whose unbelievable story was initially published by Jonathan Clemente, MD. Possibly this is because I was born and raised in the same state (Iowa) and heard many of the astonishing stories passed down about Bob's activities while attending dental school at Iowa. The memories go something like this:

Like many young boys his age growing up in central Iowa in the 1920s, Bob Moyers idolized the cowboys who came through town with the traveling rodeo. He was a precocious young man with a gift of gab and a trait of unabashed self-promotion. During his years at the University of Iowa, he could raise hell on a Saturday night and wake up early the next morning to perform his duties as a student pastor in several small towns near the university. Moyers was a man of small stature who had big ideas and a desire to see the world beyond Sidney, Iowa. What he lacked in physical height he made up for in pure force of will, personality, and grit.

Moyers was also a prolific writer and poet, but those activities were soon set aside with the approach of World War II. The United States National Archives provides the only firsthand account of an entirely new life for Moyers in occupied Greece during the World War II. But I don't want to preempt Norm's exciting narrative.

The final chapters of this book describe in painful detail the many prisoners of war who not only suffered endless torture at the hands of the enemy, but were also denied recompense from our government for time lost while in captivity. This fact was unknown by me and perhaps by many others of my age. As difficult as it may be to fully understand, the reality of war has long burdened much of this world. After reading this book, you will never forget that we have war heroes within our profession who deserve far greater recognition than has been offered in the past.

Ever since becoming Norm's editor in 1988, and having seen a steady stream of articles on orthodontic history in the *PCSO Bulletin*, *The Angle Orthodontist*, and the *American Journal of Orthodontics & Dentofacial Orthopedics*, it is clear to me that dental history has become the love of his life as well as mine.

David L. Turpin, DDS, MSD,
Former faculty member, University of Washington,
Former editor-in-Chief, *PCSO Bulletin*, *The Angle Orthodontist*, and *the American Journal of Orthodontics & Dentofacial Orthopedics* (now Editor Emeritus),
Member of Executive Committee, World Federation of Orthodontists, 2010-15, and
Honorary Scientific Advisor for WFO / 9th IOC, Yokohama, Japan

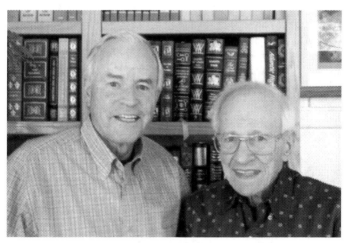

David Turpin's last visit with the
author (R.) in his home, 2014.

PREFACE

Ever since the dental officer became an integral part of the military (occurring in 1911 in the US Army), thousands of men and women of all nations have served both their profession and their country, under usually trying circumstances, diligently, and some heroically. Some lost their lives. Some were captured by the enemy and became prisoners of war (POWs), enduring beatings, starvation, and humiliation—and sometimes torture. Others volunteered for dangerous missions behind enemy lines.

I have attempted in this book to select 12 of those individuals who went beyond the line of duty to warrant special recognition. For various reasons, including information availability, I have limited my selection to (1) World War I and World War II, (2) the United States and its English-speaking allies, (3) members of the armed forces, (4) those holding a DDS or equivalent, and (5) exploits performed during wartime.

Within those limitations, What criteria to use? In the case of POWs, severity of treatment or length of servitude? Perseverance? Benefits conferred on fellow prisoners? In non-POWs, casualties inflicted? Contributions to the war effort? Perhaps some special circumstance, including postwar accomplishments, made the selectees worthy of mention. Many other candidates, not mentioned here, might qualify. To them, or their families, I offer my apologies. They will not be forgotten.

Those of you who saw the movie *They Came to Cordura* (1959) will recall that it was concerned with the travails of an Army major, Thomas Thorn (himself branded as a coward), during the 1916 US pursuit of Pancho Villa across the Mexican border. Thorn is ordered to lead a group of Medal of Honor eligibles across a barren, dangerous tract of desert, but also uses his assignment to uncover the reasons underlying their heroism, as well as to possibly redeem himself. *Cordura* was more than a Western, more than a war movie, more than a character study (although it was all of those things). It was an inquiry into three questions. The first was unspoken: What does it take to bring out the true character of a person? The answer to that question forms the essence of the plot. The second and third questions, as posed by the leading character, Major Thorn (played by Gary Cooper), were What makes a man risk his life for the common good? And, What is bravery?

Whether these questions were ever answered in the movie is left for the viewer to decide. In any case, the film inspired my own question: Can these questions be applied to someone who, only a few months previously, was comfortably peering into someone's mouth?

Bravery can be more than manning a machine gun in the face of overwhelming odds, as did our CPT Salomon. It can be venturing into uncharted territory where mutilated faces are at stake, as did our MAJ Kazanjian when he crossed the fine line between dentistry and plastic surgery. Or it can be Coenraad Moorrees administering to his fellow prisoners of war (POWs) while he himself suffered from multiple maladies.

What makes an ordinarily peace-loving dentist, when confronted with the circumstances of war, rise to the occasion and perform acts of heroism, as exemplified by these twelve dental officers, all of whom, in order to qualify for selection, needed three qualifications: (1) They had a DDS or DMD, (2) They were members of the armed forces, and (3) Their feats were performed during time of war (WWI or WWII). There was no "selection board" appointed to choose these 12. Their presence in this account was based solely on the author's opinion. To those who had relatives who they feel were overlooked, I offer my apologies.

ACKNOWLEDGMENTS

Many thanks to:

Drs Patrick K. Turley and Larry W. White, for their encouragement

Andrea Matlack of the American Dental Association, for locating hard-to-find references

Dr David L. Turpin, for writing the Foreword

Casey L. Wahl, my grandson, for being my computer geek

BOOKS BY NORMAN WAHL:

ORAL SIGNS AND SYMPTOMS
WHO WAS WHO IN ORTHODONTICS
THE GOLDEN AGE OF ORTHODONTICS

PART ONE

THE DENTIST IN THE ARMED FORCES

HISTORY OF MILITARY DENTISTRY

INTRODUCTION

IMPORTANCE OF DENTAL CARE DURING HOSTILITIES

The primary objective of the US Army Dental Corps is to help keep the fighting personnel available for action, and the commander who consistently neglects the dental health of those under his or her command can expect a decline in combat effectiveness. During World War II, recent arrivals overseas were generally in good dental condition and evacuation for dental defects was not at first critical. However, as the war progressed, some evacuation hospitals reported that a large number of men were being released from forward areas with dental problems that could have been prevented or treated on site. The resulting loss of manpower became a matter of serious concern to the leadership. Leaders also found that the ability to receive timely dental treatment had a surprising effect on morale.

1

In a survey of military mail, censors discovered that the biggest gripe expressed was not the danger of capture or the palatability of canned meat and dried eggs, but instead was the difficulty of obtaining needed dental care!

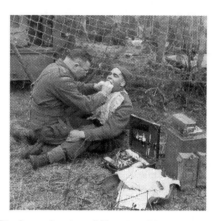

"Sit-down dentistry." Reprinted by permission of Canadian Dental Association

To ensure delivery of the best possible dental care for their personnel, commanders must first, make it possible for their dental officers to operate steadily, time after time, with the least possible interruption. Second, they must support their dental surgeons in enforcing dental appointments. Steps to improve the dental health of our fighting troops will pay important dividends in the field of battle.[1] These "fighting dentists" are all part of a continuum that began with the ancient military surgeon.

ANCIENT TIMES TO THE AMERICAN REVOLUTION

Early Military Surgery—Dentistry Before Dentists

Fifteenth- and 16th-century military surgery. The great advances being made in our knowledge of anatomy during the 15th and 16th centuries and the demands made on surgeons by the continual warfare of the period contributed to their improvement in skills. After the introduction of gunpowder in the 14th century, the wounds sustained in battle tended to increase in number and severity. Many of those practitioners who received their training on the battlefield rose to the forefront of the medical profession.

The first important treatise on military surgery, *Book of Wound Surgery*, was written by Hieronymus Brunschwig in 1497, in which he introduced a number of important techniques such as tying off blood vessels with ligatures and bringing the edges of a wound together by suturing. He was one of the first to discuss management of wounds of the mouth and surrounding tissues. He also devised a chin support for cases of jaw fracture using straps across the top of the head, and he wired patients' articulated teeth together when fragments of the mandible had been displaced.[2]

Ambroise Paré (c. 1510–December 1590) was a French barber surgeon who served in that role for kings Henry II, Francis II, Charles IX, and Henry III. Paré is considered one of the fathers of surgery and modern forensic pathology and a pioneer in surgical techniques and battlefield medicine, especially in the treatment of wounds. He was also an anatomist and the inventor of several surgical instruments. Paré was born in 1510 in Bourg-Hersent in northwestern

France. As a child he watched, and was first apprenticed to, his older brother, a barber-surgeon in Paris.

Paré was a keen observer and did not allow the beliefs of the day to supersede the evidence at hand. After completing his internship, he enlisted as a military surgeon in the army of the Duke of Montejean. It was at the Battle of Pas de Suse, his first exposure to combat, that he made his famous observation on the care of gunshot wounds. He compared one group of patients whose wounds had been treated in the traditional manner with boiling elder oil and cauterization and the remainder with a group treated with a lotion composed of egg yolk, oil of roses, and turpentine and left overnight. Paré discovered that, after a few hours, the soldiers treated with the boiling oil were in agony, whereas the ones treated with the ointment had recovered because of the antiseptic properties of turpentine. This test demonstrated the method's efficacy, and he avoided cauterization thereafter. However, treatments such as this were not widely used until many years later.

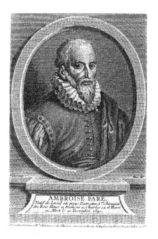

Ambroise Paré. Creative Commons.

Paré also reintroduced the ligature of arteries (first used by Galen) instead of cauterization during amputation. The usual method of sealing wounds by searing with a red-hot iron often failed to arrest the bleeding and caused patients to die of shock. For the ligature technique, he designed the *Bec de Corbeau* ("crow's beak"), a predecessor of the modern hemostat. Paré detailed the technique of using ligatures to prevent hemorrhaging during amputation in his 1564 book *Treatise on Surgery*.

During his work with injured soldiers, Paré documented the pain experienced by amputees which they perceived as sensation in the "phantom" amputated limb. Paré believed that phantom pains occur in the brain (today's medical consensus) and not in remnants of the limb. He also performed many neurosurgical procedures. Paré attributed his special interest in dental maladies to having first been a barber and tooth drawer. He, therefore, considered the treatment of dental diseases an integral part of the surgeon's responsibility.[3]

The importance of healthy teeth for fighting troops had long been recognized. John Woodall, surgeon general of the East India Company, stipulated which instruments to be included in surgical chests, which became regulation for the British Armed Forces. These included instruments for scaling, periodontics, and exodontia. Infantrymen and grenadiers from the seventeenth century and beyond were required to have good incisors to enable them to bite open cartridge cases. By 1857, army surgeons were urged to attempt to conserve teeth rather than extract them; instruments were issued for that purpose.[4]

Norman Wahl, DDS, MS, MA

THE AMERICAN REVOLUTION

The Continental Army was established on June 14, 1775, without any provision for dental care for the troops—a policy that continued until 1901: All soldiers were responsible for their own dental care. Many of General (GEN) George Washington's troops received their dental treatment at the local blacksmith's shop, often using tongs for forceps. There is an account of a blacksmith who fractured six sound teeth while attempting to extract a soldier's upper second molar.[5]

Washington himself was beset with dental problems most of his life. By 1796, he was edentulous. Two of his most well-known "plates" were the lead dentures fabricated by Charles Peale and the hippopotamus ivory dentures made by John Greenwood. Other officers went to one of the few private dentists in the vicinity or to their family physician. Midnight rider Paul Revere performed the first recorded case of forensic identification for the military when he established the identity of Major General (MG) Joseph Warren's remains on Bunker Hill because he recognized a false tooth that he had made for the general.

At that time, the French were considered the best dentists in the world. Comte de Rochambeau had two trained dentists in his navy when he arrived in Newport, Rhode Island, to support the colonial cause. One of these, Jacques (James) Gardette, provided dental care for Rochambeau's 6000-man navy and was probably the first medically trained practitioner to treat colonial soldiers.[2] He was the first to publish a scientific article on a dental topic.[7] The other, Jacques Le Mayeur, became Washington's dentist.

POSTREVOLUTION

During the War of 1812 and the Mexican War, American soldiers received needed care from civilian dentists or itinerant "tooth drawers." If no civilian source was available, ill-prepared Army physicians and hospital stewards tried to provide emergency dental care.[8] In 1844, Dr Edward Maynard, inventor of the Maynard rifle, was the first to suggest that dentists be made an official part of the military. In 1858, Dr Henry McKellops petitioned Congress to provide support for dental services in the armed forces.[8] All to no avail. Our legislators were not yet ready to recognize the need for dental care for service members.

REFERENCES FOR CHAPTER I

1   Jeffcott GF. Command responsibility for adequate dental service. *Mil Rev*. 1947;27(5):38-42.

2   Hieronymus Brunschwig. Available at: https://en.wikipedia.org/wiki/Hieronymus_Brunschwig. Accessed December 15, 2018.

3   Ambroise Paré. Available at: https://en.wikipedia.org/wiki/Ambroise_Par%C3%A9. Accessed December 21, 2018.

4   Parry C. Military dentistry: A walk through the Web sources. *Dent Hist Mag*. 2013 (autumn); 7(2):25.

5   Blinn HC. The turnkey. East Canterbury, N.H.: *The Manifesto*. Jan 1898:142.

6   Garant PR. *The Long Climb: From Barber-Surgeons to Doctors of Dental Surgery*. Chicago: Quintessence; 2013.

7   Curtis EK. Dentists at war. *J Am Col Dentists*. 1996 (Summer); 63:31.

8   King JE, Hynson RG. Highlights in the history of U.S. Army dentistry. Office of the Surgeon General. 2007. Available at: https://history.amedd.army.mil/corps/dental/general/highlights/Highlights.pdf. Accessed October 10, 2018.

US ARMY DENTISTRY TO WORLD WAR II

CIVIL WAR—UNION

There was no military dental care for soldiers in the Union Army during the Civil War. Not so in the Confederate Army (see below). Those responsible in the Union hierarchy thought so little of the dental needs of their recruits that they failed to distribute an item so basic and inexpensive as a tooth brush. This was despite protestations and petitions from the American Dental Association (ADA) and prominent dental practitioners. The condition of the teeth of the Union Army's recruits was abominable, but this was not entirely due to army life. The high rate of rejection was due to the recruits' failure to meet even the low prevailing dental standards. Even so, in 1864, nearly 10% of exemptions were dentally related. By the 1860s, three dental schools had opened in the United States, but the availability of 5000 dentists apparently had not "trickled down" to the thousands of dentally deprived recruits.

The only health-care-related personnel available to Union soldiers were medical surgeons and stewards, whose dental experience was nil. Soldiers tended to neglect basic care of their teeth, and their diet did nothing to promote dental health. In addition, dental procedures usually cost more than the typical soldier could afford. Most potential recruits were rejected if they lacked six upper and lower front teeth. These were considered necessary to bite off the ends of the cartridges used in the muzzle-loading rifles of the time. The Union's lack of proper dental care for its troops created a distinct disadvantage in terms of troop fitness.

Dr W.B. Roberts of New York suggested in a paper that a dental surgeon be assigned to each regiment along with the regular medical surgeon. He pointed out the high losses in British troops resulting from the poor condition of their soldiers' teeth, while the French army had fewer noncombat losses because of their emphasis on dental care, which included issuing tooth brushes and requiring the use thereof. Although the American Dental Convention of 1861 appealed to President Lincoln to attach a corps of dental surgeons to the Army, his acting surgeon-general failed to act on the suggestion. Dr Roberts further claimed that "the Army surgeon is not only utterly incompetent to the proper care of teeth, but he is also entirely averse to it." The Union military had a clear disadvantage as a result of its lack of dental care, and its soldiers suffered accordingly.[1]

CIVIL WAR—CONFEDERACY

In 1860, there were about 1000 dentists in the Southern states but there was no dental school or publication per se. Only about 10% of these dentists had received a formal education. As for materials, Southern dentists were almost entirely dependent on the North for their dental supplies. The only dental society had been founded in Georgia in 1859 with 11 members. By the end of 1864, dentists were required to pay for gold foil and gold plate with gold or silver currency. At that time, the price of gold foil was $64 an ounce, so the price of a gold filling was $120, and for an upper denture on a gold or vulcanite base the cost was between $1800 and $4000. To put these prices in perspective, it should be realized that a pair of shoes cost $300, cavalry boots were $1000, and that an ordinary felt hat ran from $300 to $500.[2]

The average Confederate soldier was wounded six times seriously enough to receive treatment. A large percentage of these wounds involved the face and jaws. Each soldier admitted to a hospital was given a dental examination. However, any procedures would have to be carried out with the concurrence of the attending medical officer, and the dentist would have had to provide his own instruments.[3]

At the start of the war, the United States Government declared medical and surgical instruments as contraband of war, so the Confederacy was required to furnish its own materia medica. Because of shortages, the fields and forests of the South were scoured for plants that could be used to supply quinine and other drugs.

Dentists assigned to hospitals were usually provided with a room with good lighting, hot and cold water, soap and towels, and a servant or soldier to assist. Operating chairs were made to the dentist's specifications by the hospital carpenter. Dentists were usually given the rank of hospital steward, although in some cases, they could be full surgeons with corresponding pay and benefits. A dental officer's typical day would see the preparation of 20 to 30 fillings, the extraction of 15 or 20 teeth, and the removal of limitless tartar.

One of the lessons learned from the then recent Crimean War (1854–55) was that many wounds of the face healed relatively rapidly and that compound fractures of the facial bones did not have as serious an outcome as fractures of the extremities. Surgeons learned that many wounds to the face from gunshot were usually more distressing cosmetically than they were dangerous to life.[4]

POST-CIVIL WAR—FIRST US MILITARY DENTIST

It would be 1901 before the official formation of the US Army Dental Corps, but William Saunders could lay claim to having been the Army's first official dentist. At the same time, the Corps of Cadets at West Point became the first military group to receive regular, free dental care.

The US Military Academy had employed the occasional services of visiting dentists since 1825; however, Dr Saunders was the first dentist in uniform. Having obtained his training as a dental preceptor in New York City, he was ordered to report to West Point in 1858 as a hospital steward. Saunders served the needs of that institution for 48 years. Occupying a dental room within the cadet hospital, Saunders treated, in addition to the cadets, officers, enlisted men, and civilian personnel stationed at the post.

On January 29, 1872, the academy superintendant, Colonel (COL) Thomas H. Ruger, sent the following letter to the Secretary of War: "I have the honor to request to place Hospital Steward William Saunders . . . upon special service to perform necessary dental work for Cadets . . . he is competent, and in every way an unexceptionable person to do dental work for the families of officers and professors, as for Cadets. . . ."

Saunders, who died on August 3, 1906, was the first soldier to be recognized as a United States military dentist.[5]

SPANISH-AMERICAN WAR

The War with Spain and the Philippine Insurrection had several causes, one being the growth of American imperialism and another being Cuba's growing desire for independence from Spain. But the proximate cause was the explosion and sinking of the *USS Maine* in Havana Harbor in February 1898. Among other outcomes, this war laid the foundation for the Army Dental Corps. The placing of American soldiers on foreign soil, remote from the usual sources of dental care, forced the Medical Department to recognize the need for a dental specialty.

However, less than a month after the war started, the National Dental Association introduced a bill in Congress to establish an Army Dental Corps, but it failed because the surgeon general did not back it. If the concept of a dental corps was not acceptable at the national level, then it was left to the unit commanders to take it upon themselves to see that care was provided.

As a result, a number of hospital stewards, some of whom were already dentists, were recruited to provide dental services. In 1898, soon after the start of hostilities, Dr W.H. Ware, an enlisted man, became the first dentist to be officially appointed to practice the profession of dentistry in the US Army. He was not given the title "dental surgeon," however, but instead was classified as "hospital corpsman," and was attached to the Eighth Army Convalescent Hospital in Manila.

Not long afterward, when Lieutenant Colonel (LTC) Louis Maus, chief surgeon of the Seventh Army Corps, learned that some members of the hospital corps were dentists as well as physicians, he determined to organize a department of dentistry for his unit. The result proved so successful that the surgeon general finally relented and in February 1901, an amendment to Senate Bill 4300, provided for the hiring of contract dental surgeons by the US Army, was passed. Accordingly, 30 contract dental surgeons were appointed.

In 1951, at the 50th anniversary celebration of the founding of the Army Dental Corps, COL Edwin P. Tignor, one of the 30 contract dentists, said that "Congress and the surgeon general decided to hire us as civilians first to see how it would work out and that early Army dentists were paid $150 a month—$13 a month more than first lieutenants of the Medical Corps received.[6]

PRE-WORLD WAR I

The years between the Spanish-American War and World War I (WWI) saw marked progress toward establishing a permanent dental corps. The following time line encapsulates these developments:

1. Before 1901, there had been no organized dental service for the Army. Emergency dental services were rendered by medical officers and enlisted men.
2. December 6, 1900: An amendment to Senate Bill 4300 is accepted by Congress, becoming the original law providing for contract dental surgeons.

3. February 2, 1901: An act provides for the appointment of contract dental surgeons to serve the officers and enlisted men of the Army, in the proportion of one for every 1000 persons, not to exceed 30 in all.

4. February 11, 1901: First 30 contract dental surgeons are appointed by Army surgeon general, but only nine of these may be stationed in the United States. They will wear the uniform and have the privileges of an Army officer, but hold no rank. One of these 30 is Dr John S. Marshall, outstanding dentist, author of several textbooks, and organizer of Northwestern Dental School.

5. April 20, 1906: Dr Leonie von Meusebach-Zasch is the first woman dentist to work for the Army when she was hired to support emergency relief for victims of the San Francisco earthquake. William A. Birch is believed to be the first African American steward-dentist to be commissioned in the US Army Dental Corps.

6. 1906: That same year, the ADA establishes a Committee on Army and Navy Legislation to elevate the status of military dentistry.

7. April 23, 1908: Recognition by law of the contract dental surgeon as part of the Army Medical Department.

8. March 3, 1911: An act is passed providing for a Dental Corps consisting of dental surgeons in the proportion of one to 1000 of the enlisted strength of the Army.

9. Raids by Pancho Villa along the US-Mexican border in 1916 result in deployment of both active and National Guard officers and create an awareness that dentists still lack operational field

skills, military administrative knowledge, and trauma-related training—requirements in dental preparedness that are unique to military service.

10. September 1916: The Army establishes its first dental training school at Fort Bliss, Texas.

11. October 6, 1917: Officials determine that officers of the Army Dental Corps are to receive the same rank, pay, promotions, and retirement benefits as Army Medical Corps officers.[7,8,13]

WORLD WAR I

The outbreak of World War I caught most armies unprepared, without adequate—if any—contingent to serve the dental needs of their personnel. For instance, the British Expeditionary Force had no dentists at war's start and less than 1000 at the end of the conflict. When war with Germany broke out on April 6, 1917, the strength of the US Army Dental Corps was 86 officers on active duty (it reached 4620 by November 1918). Fortunately, Congress had passed the National Defense Act of 1916, which included reorganization of the Army Dental Corps and abolishing the probationary contract system. It also permitted immediate commissioning of dental officers as first lieutenants (1LTs) with advancement to captain (CPT) after 8 years and to major (MAJ) after 24 years of active service.[9] In August 1917, the first dental unit of the American Expeditionary Forces (AEF) arrived in France.

Trench warfare in World War I saw a high incidence of facial trauma, creating a great demand for oral surgeons and dentists with experience in reconstructive prosthodontics. Raising the head and neck above the trench line resulted in certain disfigurement or death from enemy fire. The enormous number of jaw fracture cases was described by Francis Wilson, chief of the American Ambulance Hospital at Juilly, France:

> In September 1915, I had 52 cases of fracture of the maxillae enter the hospital in one afternoon; of these, I saw only two completely cured—all the others were sent to hospitals away from the war zone some 10 days later. Among these 52 cases were some of the worst that have ever come under my observation . . . one poor fellow had the entire face below the eyes blown off, nothing remaining of the inferior maxilla. . . . my work was to wire these [pieces of bone] together so that the man could eat soft food besides being more comfortable.[10]

It was left to Varaztad Kazanjian (1879–1974) to develop modern techniques of plastic surgery for battlefield wounds (see section on Kazanjian below). In the meantime, more personnel and more training were clearly needed. On August 9, 1917, MAJ William G. Logan, MD, DDS, a Medical Corps Reserve officer, was appointed chief of the newly created Dental Section, Personnel Division, Office of the Surgeon General and first Chief, Army Dental Corps. As such, he substantially increased the size of the Dental Reserve, organized maxillofacial surgical teams, and established dental officer basic training and an enlisted dental assistant training program at Fort Oglethorpe, Georgia. In September 1916, the Army established its first dental training school at Fort Bliss, Texas. In addition, the War Department conducted a student Army and Navy Training Corps at all dental schools approved by the Surgeon General.[11]

On November 15, 1917, the curriculum of the Army Sanitary School in France was expanded to include courses in approved methods of war dentistry procedures, surgery of the face and jaws, first aid for the gassed and wounded, transportation of the wounded, and administration of serum and general anesthesia.

Any ideas that newly minted dental officers were in for a life of glamour and excitement was soon dispelled upon their induction. Typical was the experience of Dr Sheridan C. Waite. Upon graduating from the University of Buffalo School of Dental Medicine in 1918, Waite enlisted as a member of Dental Company No. 1, the only company in the world consisting of only dentists. On his arrival at Camp Greenleaf, Fort Oglethorpe, Georgia, Waite was billeted with other members of the company in a stable. Waite recalled:

> Mules were removed from two long, narrow stables and the ground was given a good cleaning. Folding cots were lined up in a row on the dirt floor and covered with straw mattresses with a heavy blanket—no sheets. Along the open side of the stable was hung a heavy tarpaulin that could be rolled up during the clear days. The cots were aired out in the sun to prevent us from catching the flu.[12]

Before long, Waite became part of the select group of dental officers who, from July 1917 to May 1919, treated almost a million-and-a-half patients, placing a like number of restorations, and performing over 380,000 extractions and a comparable number of prosthetic units at a cost of seven officers and seven enlisted assistants killed. Thirty-six dentists and assistants were wounded in combat and eight dental officers died of disease.[13]

REFERENCES FOR CHAPTER II

1   Dammann GE. Dental care during the Civil War. *Ill Dent J.* 1984;53:12-17.

2   Schwartz LL. War problems of dentistry: the South in the Civil War. *J Am Dent Assoc.*1945;32:37-42.

3   Tebo HG. Oral surgery in the Confederate Army. *Bul Hist Dent.* 1976;24:28-35.

4   Civil War dentistry. Available at: https://ehistory.osu.edu/topics/uscw. Accessed October 14, 2019.

5   Hyson JM. William Saunders: the United States Army's first dentist—West Point's forgotten man. *Mil Med.* 1984(August);19-23.

6   The Spanish-American War, 1898— AMEDD Center and School. Available at: https://ke.army.mil › bordeninstitute › other_pub › dental › DCchapter05. Accessed July 5, 2018.

7   Army Extension Courses, Special Text No. 51, Dental Administration. Washington, DC: Government Printing Office, 1939.

8   Neel S. Historical highlights of the Army Dental Corps. U.S. Army Health Services Command. San Antonio, Texas: Fort Sam Houston, 1974:3-10.

9   Curtis EK. Dentists at war. *J Am Col Dentists.* 1996;63(summer):31-33.

10   Hyson JM. Army dental history. Available at: https://history.amedd.army.mil/corps/dental/dental.html. n.d. Accessed June 16, 2018.

11   King JE, Hynson RG. Highlights in the history of U.S. Army dentistry. Office of the Surgeon General. 2007. Available at: https://history.amedd.army.mil/corps/dental/general/highlights/Highlights.pdf. Accessed October 10, 2018.

12   Waite SC. Looking for Dental Company No. 1. *The Bridge.* Chicago: Northwestern University Dental School; 1988.

13   Hyson JM. Army dental history. Accessed September 8, 2018.

US ARMY DENTISTRY—
WWII TO POST-VIETNAM

WORLD WAR II

Status of dental officers. When the United States entered
World War II (WWII) on December 7, 1941, the Army had
316 active duty dental officers and a Reserve Corps of 2589.
Each Army division had an average of 50 dental officers.
The goal was to have a ratio of about 1 to 312 (infantry)
and 1 to 487 (armor). Yet, Army procurement officials were
concerned that the Dental Corps would be understaffed
because of the recent Depression, current rigorous dental
school entrance requirements, and the decline in the dental
population of the United States in the late '30s by 8000 since
the prior decade.

Despite their performance in World War I, dentists
were initially drafted as privates, but thanks to the Army
Specialized Training Program (ASTP) and the Navy V-12
Program, dental students were guaranteed commissions on
graduation.[1] The newly created Army Dental Corps had to
deal with gigantic troop recruitment, making up their lack

of staff by the massive training of Army dentists in close cooperation with America's dental schools and by signing up many civilian dentists.

At the war's onset, there was considerable professional rivalry between officers of the medical and dental corps. Physicians regarded dentists (already fighting for recognition) as upstarts in the health care field who claimed that dental treatment would cure an individual's medical problems (so said the MDs). The main points of resentment held by the dentists, however, were (1) not being able to present their views and recommendations directly to their commanders and (2) oral health care being dispensed in physician-controlled facilities because dental officers were not allowed to command these facilities. The dental surgeon was only an advisor to the surgeon, without final authority—even in the dental clinic. Thus, the dental officer had a much lower chance of achieving field grade (major and above). It was not until June 1945 that the command privileges enjoyed by other Army officers were extended to dental officers. Finally, on March 17, 1946, Thomas L. Smith became the first dental officer to achieve the permanent rank of major general when he was appointed chief of the Dental Corps in March 1938, Leigh C. Fairbank, an orthodontist, had become the first dental officer to reach general officer rank when he was promoted to brigadier general (BG) and appointed eighth chief of the Army Dental Corps.

Norman Wahl, DDS, MS, MA

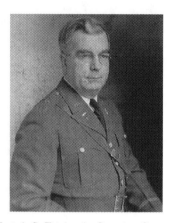

BG Leigh S. Fairbank. Creative Commons.

Dentists as medical officers. In addition to providing the usual dental services, such as fillings, extractions, and prosthetics, the Army dental officer could be called upon to undertake the role of paymaster, sanitary inspector, mess officer, or whatever duty was required by the commanding officer.[2] In a combat situation, he was likely to find himself taking on the function of a medical officer.

When a dental officer was assigned to a tactical organization, his primary duty was that of a battalion or regimental dental surgeon, but he was also an assistant to the surgeon in an advisory capacity on dental matters. In combat, he was an assistant battalion surgeon, in which case he could be called upon to take charge of a battalion aid station charged with rendering first aid and assisting the medical department in the evacuation of battlefield casualties. Therefore, it was essential that he be familiar with the evacuation procedures of the tactical organization to which he was assigned. It was mandatory that he be trained in administering first aid and providing treatment for shock, chemical burns, and the use of arm and leg splints.[3]

Progression of evacuees with maxillofacial injuries.
Within a few minutes after receiving his wound, the injured
man was usually picked up by a *company aid man* (medic) of
his own organization. Although this Medical Department
soldier was trained in first aid so he could stop bleeding or
take whatever emergency steps were necessary to save life,
his principal function was to get the casualty into the hands
of a supporting medical unit that would remove him from
the combat area. The aid man stopped hemorrhage, applied
bandages, and directed the wounded man to the *battalion
aid station* several hundred yards to the rear. If the patient
could not walk, he was carried by litter bearers.

Because the battalion aid station had only limited
facilities and was poorly protected from enemy fire, the
wounded man was held there only long enough to prepare
him for further evacuation and to arrange for transportation
to the rear. His bandages might be adjusted, he might be
given plasma or a sedative if necessary, and his airway was
checked, but as soon as possible he was transferred to litter
bearers who had been sent forward from a *collecting station*.
These collecting stations were normally established within
litter-carrying distance of the battalion aid stations and, if
possible, on a passable motor road to the rear. Two medical
officers were available, having somewhat more elaborate
equipment allowing them to attempt emergency procedures
that were not feasible at the aid stations. The collecting
station was still within easy range of hostile artillery
and mortar fire, however, so its primary mission was the
assembly and evacuation of patients rather than treatment.
In the absence of a dental officer at the collecting station,
the maxillofacial patient usually received only such general
care as would permit further transportation by ambulance
to *the clearing station*.

Division clearing stations with four medical officers and at least one dental officer were normally established several miles behind the lines for further assembly and treatment of patients from the collecting stations. Typically, a clearing station included a small operating room and ward tents for the temporary care of patients who could not immediately be removed to a hospital. Clearing station staff had to be ready to move on short notice so that only the most urgent operational procedures were performed. A maxillofacial injury normally received little care at this point beyond the control of bleeding, treatment of shock, and possibly the temporary immobilization of fractured jaws with some type of bandage. As soon as possible following such emergency treatment, the patient was removed by ambulance to an *evacuation hospital*, where nontransportable maxillofacial patients were cared for. Here he was placed under the care of a maxillofacial team, usually consisting of an oral surgeon, a plastic surgeon, and the necessary nurses and technicians. In this installation could be found three dental officers, two portable operating units, and one portable laboratory unit.[4] Next in the chain was the *general hospital*, which usually remained a fixed installation throughout the period of combat. Here could be found five dental officers who ideally had wide experience in surgical and operative procedures including extensive maxillofacial repair, using splints and other prosthetic devices.

Patients needing prolonged treatment or recuperation were transferred to *medical centers or convalescent hospitals* where dental officers of all specialties were on duty and prepared to perform appropriate permanent work.[4]

Of more than 18,000 dentists serving during World War II, 20 lost their lives in enemy action, 10 died in captivity, and 81 succumbed to disease and nonbattle injuries.

KOREAN WAR (JUNE 1950—JULY 1953)

On June 25, 1950, North Korea invaded its neighbor, South Korea. By the following day, President Harry S. Truman had authorized the use of US forces in the ensuing conflict. The following March, Dr. Helen E. Myers became the first woman to serve as an Army dental officer, entering with the rank of CPT.

The Korean War saw the introduction of area dental support (as opposed to unit dental support). This concept would evolve into the KJ Detachment of the Vietnam War era, the HA Detachment of the early 1970s, and the dental company of the post-1991 Gulf War era.

The peak strength of the Army Dental Corps during the Korean War was 2641 officers, 370 of whom served in the Koreas, two dental officers were killed, and one was declared dead after being classed as missing in action.[5]

VIETNAM WAR

Although the beginning and ending dates for the involvement of the US Army in the Vietnam War are arguable, the US Military Assistance Advisory Group (MAAG) was established as early as August 1950. A time line follows:

1956: The Army Dental Corps enters the picture when LTC (later, BG) Jack P. Pollock is assigned on a temporary duty (TDY) status to MAAG as dental advisor for the team.

December 1, 1956: BG James M. Epperly is promoted to MG and appointed as the 13th chief of the Army Dental Corps.

August 10, 1957: The WWII-type of temporary building is replaced by a modern, air-conditioned dental unit in Fort Dix, NJ, and elsewhere, built exclusively for dentistry.

August 1, 1960: COL Joseph L. Bernier is promoted to BG and sworn in as the 14th chief of the Army Dental Corps. His accomplishments will include (1) while in the service, installing an Army-wide preventive dentistry program, (2) following his discharge, applying the same program in civilian practice, and (3) organizing oral pathology as a dental specialty.

April 18, 1962: The first dental unit—the 36th Medical Detachment (Dental Service)—is the first dental unit to deploy, as well as the first of the KJ Detachment type that was originally fielded at the end of the Korean War. The old electric motor, belt-driven handpieces, and fixed-position, tubular canvas chairs are replaced with stateside-type fixed equipment, and a compressed-air, rotor-handpiece system, developed specifically for field military use, is installed, creating the modern, mobile capability required for operational support.[5]

November 15, 1967: BG Robert B. Shira is promoted to MG and appointed 15th chief, Army Dental Corps (by then having 2656 officers). After General Shira visited Viet Nam in the spring of 1968 and heard the commanders' complaints about soldiers being taken off duty because of dental emergencies, major improvements in mission support occurred: (1) a 20% increase in dental officer strength; (2) increased availability of field dental equipment; (3) enactment of the Dental Combat Effectiveness Program (DCEP); (4) use of an improved intermediate restorative material (IRM) to avoid unnecessary extractions; (5) field screening and continuing care at theater in-processing and at forward troop sites in Vietnam; (6) mass application of self-applied 9% fluoride paste. Dr Shira later became dean of Tufts University School of Dental Medicine and president of the ADA.

July 1969: Withdrawal of dental units begins.

February 12, 1973: The last dental unit, the 38th Medical Detachment is inactivated.

The largest number of dental officers on active duty during the Vietnam War was 2817, but only a maximum of 290 were stationed in Vietnam at any one time. The concept of support was a combination of unit support (one dentist per brigade), hospital support (usually one oral surgeon per hospital), and area support (14 dental service units and one dental command and control unit). Four Army dental officers and four dental enlisted soldiers lost their lives in the Vietnam War.[6]

POST-VIETNAM

Under the leadership of MG Edwin H. Smith, Army Dental Service chief from 1971–75, there were improvements in management, workload reporting and analysis, and the use of dental therapy assistants (DTAs), among others.

After a career as chief of oral pathology, director of the US Army Institute of Dental Research, and director of medical personnel, MG Surindar N. Bhaskar, was sworn in as the 17th chief of the Army Dental Corps. MG Bhaskar played a major role in the Army's separating its dental from its medical services to improve dental care. In 1976, he testified before the House of Representatives that dental funds were being "mischanneled and misused." Together with MG Smith, he was instrumental in separating the US Army Dental Activity (DENTAC) from the hospital and medical activity. Gen Bhaskar was the only dental chief who was board certified in both oral pathology and oral medicine, as well as having completed a residency in periodontics. Among his many publications was the widely read *Synopsis of Oral Pathology*.

As the Gulf War escalated in 1990, MG Bill B. Lefler guided Army dentistry through hectic mobilization and deployment. While Desert Storm, Hurricane Andrew, and Restore Home (Somalia peacekeeping) stretched dental capabilities, the Army dental care system underwent one of the most turbulent periods of Army restructuring in Army history. In 1994, the US Army Dental Command (DENCOM) was established to maximize efficiency in serving soldiers and their commanders. Corrective measures (such as special pay, a scholarship program, and use of civilian manpower) were undertaken in the late 1990s to address a severe manpower shortage.[6]

REFERENCES FOR CHAPTER III

1   Curtis EK. Dentists at war. *J Am Col Dentists*. 1996;63(summer):31-33.

2   Gillett MC. *The Army Medical Department, 1917-1941*. Washington DC: Center of Military History, United States Army, 2009.

3   The Evacuation of Maxillofacial Casualties. Available at: https://history.amedd.army.mil/booksdocs/wwii/dental/ch8.htm. Accessed October 2, 2018.

4   Clopper PW. The place and duties of the dentist in the Army and Navy. *Ill Dent J*. 1943;12:333-335.

5   U.S. Army Medical Department. Office of Medical History. Korean War and Vietnam War. Available at: https://www.google.com/search?sxsrf=ACYBGNT . . . Accessed October 18, 2018.

6   King JE, Hynson RG. Highlights in the history of U.S. Army dentistry. Office of the Surgeon General. 2007. Available at https://history.amedd.army.mil/corps/dental/general/highlights/Highlights.pdf. Accessed October 10, 2018.

IV

DENTISTRY IN OTHER SERVICES

US NAVY DENTISTRY

Pre-World War I. On 22 August 1912, the 62nd Congress established the US Navy Dental Corps. The Secretary of the Navy was authorized to appoint no more than 30 acting assistant dental surgeons to be a part of the Medical Department.

In October 1912, Emory Bryant and William Cogan were the first two dental officers to enter active duty with the US Navy. In 1916, Congress authorized the president to appoint and commission dental surgeons in the Navy at the rate of one dentist per 1000 enlisted personnel.[1]

World War I. During World War I, the Surgeon General of the United States mandated that dental officers complete a 10-week course in advanced oral surgery at Naval Station Great Lakes. The Corps expanded from 35 to over 500. With America's involvement in World War I, the Navy deployed dental officers on combatant ships and with Marine ground combat units. The first dental officer stationed on a ship was LTJG Carl Ziesel, aboard the transport USS *Leviathan*.

Two dental officers were awarded the Medal of Honor for their heroic actions while serving with the Marines in France: LTJG Alexander Lyle with the 5th Marine Regiment and LTJG Weedon Osborne (posthumously) with the 6th Marine Regiment during the advance on Bourches, France.

Early in 1922, the Dental Division in the Bureau of Medicine and Surgery was created. Shortly after February 3, 1923, the U.S. Naval Dental School opened as the dental department of the United States Naval Medical School. Its purpose was to furnish postgraduate instruction in dental medicine to officers of the Dental Corps of the Navy and to train and equip men of the Hospital Corps as assistants to dental officers. There were 150 dental officers on duty at the time.

During this era, Navy Dentistry began to focus heavily on prevention of disease, which was a unique approach at the time and remains a quality that distinguishes the Corps today. Navy dentists demonstrated their skills throughout the 1920s and 1930s in Navy and Marine operations in such places as Haiti, Nicaragua, and China. By 1939, 255 dental officers served at 22 major dental facilities ashore and afloat. Among them was the hospital ship USS *Relief.*[2]

World War II. Two Navy Dental Corps officers were killed and four were wounded in the attack on Pearl Harbor in 1941; they would not be the last dental officers to die in the line of duty. As the US prepared for world conflict, Navy dentistry's active duty numbers swelled to its highest levels ever—ultimately reaching 7000 dental officers and 11,000 dental technicians. Active in nearly every engagement during the war, dental personnel who were assigned to operational units in the South Pacific often assisted in emergency medical operations ashore, especially facial trauma cases requiring surgery. Numerous dental officers were killed in action aboard warships and in major battles in Guadalcanal, Tarawa, Saipan, and Iwo Jima. For their heroic efforts, 93 dental officers received personal awards, including the Silver Star, the Legion of Merit, the Navy and Marine Corps Medal, and the Bronze Star Medal.

By 1943, more than 3500 dentists were serving on active duty. In June 1944, the first woman dentist in the armed forces, Lieutenant (LT) Sara Krout, DC, USNR, reported to Naval Station Great Lakes, IL. She remained in the Navy Reserves after the war and retired as a commander in 1961.

In February 1945, the first self-contained mobile dental treatment unit began operation. Mobile units were developed to provide dental treatment to small groups of naval personnel in isolated areas or at pierside, a practice common today in many fleet support areas. As the value of taking dental capabilities to the fleet became more popular, plans were authorized in August 1945 to build four dental clinic ships, but these plans were canceled when the war ended. At the time of the Japanese surrender, there were 1545 dental clinics in operation, with 459 dental officers at the Navy's largest clinic at Great Lakes alone.[3]

Post-World War II. During this period, the Naval Dental College was commanded by CAPT George W. "Bill" Ferguson, DDS, who played a significant role in the desegregation of the military, creation of the State of Israel, and the promotion of sit-down dentistry and expanded duties of dental auxiliaries.[3]

Korean War. On 27 June 1950, President Harry S. Truman ordered the US Armed Forces into action in Korea. As the 1st Marine Division deployed, dental officers and technicians marched onto the battlefield, providing dental and medical support at forward locations. Korea marked the first time in history that enlisted men of the Navy wore dental rating badges into combat. One such man was Dentalman Thomas A. Christianson, who was awarded the Navy Cross posthumously for his gallant efforts while serving with the 1st Amphibious Tractor Battalion.

At the peak of the war, 1900 dental officers and 4700 dental technicians were on active duty. As in both world wars, dental personnel served heroically. Fifteen dental officers earned personal commendations, including the Silver Star, the Bronze Star, and the Navy and Marine Corps Commendation Ribbon with Combat V.[3]

Vietnam War. By the beginning of the '60s, Navy dentistry operated from 160 shore-based facilities and aboard 156 ships. To support Marine Corps operations, the Navy developed innovative ways to use their skills in the field. Able to deploy nine mobile dental units on trailers, they also developed more powerful rotary instruments and a field x-ray and developing unit.

These field dental capabilities proved their worth when a detachment of the 3rd Dental Company deployed with Marines to Vietnam in June 1965. Many more dental teams would follow. Between 1965 and 1973, Dental Corps personnel from the 1st, 3rd, and 11th Dental Companies, along with detachments of the 15th Dental Company, deployed to Vietnam in support of Marine ground and air combat units. In addition to caring for Marines, dental personnel participated in many civic action programs rendering humanitarian aid to Vietnamese civilians. They were also busy participating in the training of Vietnamese dentists in basic and advanced dental procedures, as part of the Vietnamization program.

At the peak of the Vietnam War, there were 420 dental officers and 790 dental technicians (approximately one-fifth of the Dental Corps) deployed with Marine units.[3]

Post-Vietnam. In 1975, the nuclear-powered aircraft carrier, USS *Nimitz* was commissioned. The *Nimitz* had the most advanced and capable dental facility afloat, supporting seven dental operating rooms, a prosthetic laboratory, a central sterilization room, an x-ray suite, and a preventive dentistry room. When a Navy jet crashed on the *Nimitz* flight deck on 26 May 1981, killing 14 and injuring 48, dental personnel were an integral asset to the mass casualty response and the overall team effort.

On October 23, 1983, the bombing of the Marine headquarters and barracks of Battalion Landing Team 1/8 of the 24th Marine Amphibious Unit at Beirut International Airport, Lebanon, left 241 American servicemen dead. The only on-scene Navy physician was killed, along with 18 Navy hospital corpsmen. Two dental officers assigned to the 24th Marine Amphibious Unit coordinated emergency trauma care with 15 hospital corpsmen, treating 65 casualties in the first two hours following the explosion. LTs Bigelow and Ware would later be awarded Bronze Stars for their leadership and emergency medical services. Additional dental personnel aboard the USS *Iwo Jima* joined medical teams ashore to provide care and support for survivors.

In July 1984, the Navy began conversion of two supertankers to hospital ships. The USNS *Mercy* and the USNS *Comfort* were placed into service in December 1986. With 1000 beds and 12 operating rooms, each ship could provide comprehensive dental services in two operating rooms, four dental treatment rooms, and a dental laboratory. More recently, when the four battleships—*Iowa*, *New Jersey*, *Missouri*, and *Wisconsin*—were recommissioned, dental spaces were upgraded to provide high quality dental support.

Navy dentistry supported Marine deployments in Kuwait (1990), Somalia (1992), and Port-au-Prince, Haiti

(1998; humanitarian assistance was provided, as well). After the terrorist attacks on the World Trade Center, on September 11, 2001, Tri-service Branch Dental Clinic personnel were among the first responders to the carnage. Without regard for personal safety, five members ran into the burning building to save lives, while others began initial triage and treatment of the injured.[3]

Today, through Operation Enduring Freedom and Operation Iraqi Freedom, the Navy Dental Corps continues to maintain high operational readiness. The dental community is aggressively integrating with both the medical and the line communities to prepare for the latest challenge, Homeland Defense. They deploy routinely with Marine expeditionary units and aboard ships, where beyond their dental duties, they assume roles in triage and surgical support at Marine battalion aid stations and battle dressing stations. In addition, dental personnel continue to play a significant role in peacekeeping and nation-building through humanitarian assistance and disaster relief missions in third world countries.[3]

US AIR FORCE DENTISTRY

The first dentist to serve in the US Army Air Corps was George R. Kennebeck, who was conscripted into the Army in 1917 and commissioned as a 1LT. Although stationed Stateside during the war, he was ordered to Vladivostok the following year, where he participated in the ill-fated military intervention in Siberia launched to assist the White Russians against the Bolsheviks.

At that time, the main concern of aviation dentistry was associated with the hazards of broken or lost prosthetic appliances during flight, such as loss, breakage, and swallowing. There were also concerns about the effect of decreased oxygen levels on gum tissue as well as an increase in periodontal abscesses among aviation personnel. The introduction of high-altitude flying in the late 1930s, notably the B-17 (Flying Fortress), brought a focus on the problems of flying in the stratosphere, in particular, that poorly restored teeth ache at 25,000 feet. It was obvious that the Army Air Corps needed to evaluate these problems with the assistance of dental experts. Accordingly, in June 1942, a dental section within the office of the Air Surgeon, with LTC George R. Kennebeck as deputy, was created. Thus began the Air Force Dental Service.[4]

The problem of "aerodontalgia" was magnified with the development of the B-29 (Superfortress) in 1942. Although research on the effects of low barometric pressure on oral structures revealed no new dental pathology, 1% to 3% of airmen still experienced aerodontalgia—tooth pain resulting from lowered barometric pressure—such pain was at times severe enough to require aborting the mission. Most cases were due to preexisting sinus conditions, untreated dental pathology, or faulty dental treatment.

In time, pressurized aircraft and flying suits helped lower the incidence of "barodontalgia," as it was coming to be called. Fortunately, the gingiva was not affected by low atmospheric pressure. Not until the 1970s was it established that a major cause of barodontalgia was multirooted teeth with partial vitality. At the beginning of World War II, Air Corps dentistry, was, as with dentistry in the other services, delivered under primitive conditions. The Corps' 400 dentists had to work with World War I-vintage equipment. COL Kennebeck's experiences in 1942 Guadalcanal were typical. Often working within the range of enemy machine guns and mortars, "we had to improvise everything," he reported. "Extractions and setting of fractured jaws had to be done by feel as we had no x-rays. The old-fashioned pump pedal may have been a blessing since we didn't have electricity."[5]

It was in the field of forensic dentistry, however, that Army Air Corps dentists made some of their most significant contributions: identifying severely mutilated bodies. Dentists from the Eighth Air Force expanded on existing forms with a more detailed Flying Personnel Dental Identification Form that all air crews were required to complete. As a result, many bodies that might have gone unnamed were positively identified.

Despite these achievements, however, the morale of the rank-and-file dental officer at the close of the war was low, resulting in a mass exodus from active duty. By the end of 1946, more than 95% of dental personnel had left the Army. Three factors were suggested as being detrimental to morale: (1) an unfavorable promotion policy, (2) the perception that the Dental Corps was dominated by MDs, and (3) "amalgam lines" and other mass-production practices. Even after a separate US Air Force Dental Corps was established in 1949, only 40% of the dental officers in the Air Force were above the rank of CPT. Finally, 2 years later, the Air Force Organization Act of 1951 created "the Dental Service within the USAF as a separate service" and determining that "its activities prescribe that professional control, supervision, and staff representation be through dental personnel."[6]

Before the Korean War, dental teams were organically attached to units (unit support program). During the war, the idea of *area* support was inaugurated (as with other services). Among other changes, it placed dental facilities in higher quality, fixed facilities farther away from the front lines. Other events of note:

1953: Raya Rachlin is the first woman to be commissioned an Air Force dentist.

1957: Guidelines for aerospace dentistry are issued by the Surgeon General's office wherein the Air Force Dental Service is charged to provide "optimum dental care to the space pilots, as well as finding a way to provide dental care during prolonged space flight."

Early 1960s: The School of Aerospace Medicine is transferred to Brooks AFB, Texas, where Air Force dentists undertake the dental support of the nation's manned space program.

1960s: Dr. Ira L. Shannon, dental consultant for the Johnson Space Center, develops an edible tooth paste, NASAdent, that is foamless and can be swallowed after use—a necessity in a zero-gravity situation where normal expectoration is taboo.

1971: Air Force dentists break the "colonel barrier": promotions above LTC allowed.

1970s–80s: It is not long before Air Force forensic dentists have a chance to put their work to the test in four mass disasters (two aeronautical): Tenerife, Spain; Beirut, Lebanon; Gander, Newfoundland; and Jonestown, Guyana.

November 18, 1979: American evangelical cult leader Jim Jones leads his flock in a mass suicide ritual at Jonestown, an American colony in Guyana, in which 918 people died. COL Kenton Hartman, Air Force oral pathologist, who worked on identifying the bodies, said that, within a week, the victims' flesh "had turned into a pastelike compound; it looked like mud. The odor was just horrendous . . . and maggots were a huge problem."

1980s: 10% of the members of the Air Force Dental Service are women.

1998: Susan J. Smythe is the first woman to be appointed to a command dental surgeon position (at Space Command, Peterson AFB, Colorado).

2014: MG Roosevelt Allen is first African American assistant surgeon general for dental services.[6]

US COAST GUARD DENTISTRY

The dental needs of the Coast Guard are provided by the United States Public Health Service (USPHS) Commissioned Corps.

USPHS DENTISTRY

The Public Health Service Commissioned Corps had its beginnings with the creation of the Marine Hospital Fund in 1798, which later was reorganized in 1871 as the Marine Hospital Service and charged with the care and maintenance of merchant sailors. But as the country grew, so did the ever-expanding mission of the service. The Marine Hospital Service soon began taking on new expanding health roles that included such health initiatives to protect the commerce and health of America. One such role was quarantine.

John Maynard Woodworth, a famous surgeon in the Union Army, is credited with the formal creation of the Commissioned Corps. Woodworth organized the Marine Hospital Service medical personnel along Army military structure lines in 1889 to facilitate a mobile force of health professionals that could be relocated in response to the needs of the service and country. He established appointment standards and designed the Marine Hospital Service symbol of a fouled anchor and caduceus. Later that year, President Grover Cleveland signed into law an act that formally established the modern Public Health Service Commissioned Corps. At first open only to physicians, over the course of the twentieth century, the Corps was expanded to include 11 careers in a wide range of specialties to include dentists, among other allied health professionals.[6]

REFERENCES FOR CHAPTER IV

1   Schaffer RG. The Navy Dental Corps: 75 years of excellence. *Navy Med*. 1987(Jul-Aug);78(4):12-19.

2   Zimmerman DJ. A history of the U.S. Navy Dental Corps. Available at: https://www.defensemedianetwork.com/stories/a-history-of-the-u-s-navy-dental-corps/. Accessed July 28, 2018.

3   United States Navy Dental Corps. Available at: https://en.wikipedia.org/wiki/United_States_Navy_Dental_Corps. Accessed August 3, 2018.

4   Savage DK. 50th commemorative anniversary of the United States Air Force Dental Service, 1949-1999. Bolling AFB, DC: Office of the Assistant Surgeon General for Dental Services, United States Air Force; 1999.

5   Zimmerman DJ. A history of high-flying dental care. Available at: https://www.defensemedianetwork.com/stories/air-force-dental-service/. Accessed December 6, 2018.

6   Garvin J. USPHS Dental Category turns 100. *J Am Dent Assoc*. Available at: https://en.m.wikipedia.org/wiki/United_States_Public_Health_Service_Commissioned_Corps. Accessed October 21, 2019.

V

POWS OF US WARS TO WWII

BACKGROUND

The earliest recorded usage of the phrase "prisoner of war" dates back to 1660. For most of human history, depending on the culture of the victors, enemy combatants on the losing side in a battle who had surrendered and been taken as prisoners of war (POWs) could expect to be either slaughtered or enslaved.

The prevailing military code prescribed that warriors should prefer death over dishonor, so captured soldiers were viewed with contempt. POWs, if not murdered outright, were used as slaves or tortured or maimed for entertainment. In 352 BC, Philip of Macedon ordered 3000 prisoners from the Greek city-state of Phocos to be drowned. Romans threw prisoners into the Coliseum to die in mock battles or be eaten by wild animals. In the Dark Ages, brutality was the norm, as for example, when the Crusaders murdered 2500 Muslim prisoners during the 1105 AD siege of Acre.

However, examples of humane behavior can be found. In the fourth century AD, Bishop Acacius of Amida, touched by the plight of Persian prisoners captured in a recent war with the Roman Empire, who were held in his town under appalling conditions and destined for a life of slavery, took the initiative in ransoming them by selling his church's precious gold and silver vessels and allowing them return to their own country. During the Third Crusade (1189–92) Saladin, the sultan of Syria and Egypt, permitted the Knight Hospitaliers of Jerusalem to treat wounded Christian prisoners. By the mid-1700s, when Great Britain and France were fighting the Seven Years' War, prisoner exchange was common.[1]

We owe it to Henri Dunant, a Swiss businessman and writer, for the spur that led to the first codified international treaty addressing the welfare of the sick and wounded soldiers on the battlefield and, eventually, prisoners of war. Dunant was so shocked by the lack of facilities, personnel, and medical aid available for wounded soldiers after the Battle of Solferino in 1859, that he wrote a book, *A Memory of Solferino* (1862), on the horrors of war. His powerful message led to the establishment of the Red Cross in Geneva and the 1864 Geneva Convention. In recognition of both these accomplishments, Dunant became corecipient of the first Nobel Peace Prize in 1901. Since then, there have been three treaties and three additional protocols addressing these issues, and almost every nation on earth has signed the Geneva Conventions.[2]

Conventions

In diplomacy, the term *convention* does not have its common meaning as an assembly of people. Rather, it is used to mean *an international agreement,* or treaty.

The Geneva Conventions are rules that apply only in times of armed conflict and that seek to protect people who are not or are no longer taking part in hostilities; these include the sick and wounded of armed forces on the field, wounded, sick, and shipwrecked members of armed forces at sea, prisoners of war, and civilians. The first convention dealt with the treatment of wounded and sick armed forces in the field. The second convention dealt with the sick, wounded, and shipwrecked members of armed forces at sea. The third convention dealt with the treatment of prisoners of war during times of conflict. The fourth convention dealt with the treatment of civilians and their protection during wartime.

With respect to prisoners of war, the following acts are and shall remain prohibited at any time and in any place whatsoever:

> Violence to life and person, in particular murder of all kinds, mutilation, cruel treatment, and torture; Taking of hostages; Outrages upon dignity, in particular, humiliating and degrading treatment; and The passing of sentences and the carrying out of executions without previous judgment pronounced by a regularly constituted court, affording all the judicial guarantees which are recognized as indispensable by civilized peoples. The wounded and sick shall be collected and cared for.[3]

POWS IN US WARS

American Revolution (1775-1783)

The British expected to achieve a quick victory over the colonists, so did not anticipate the necessity of maintaining facilities for the care and feeding of prisoners. Furthermore, since they did not recognize the colonists' independence, they considered POWs to be traitors and pirates. The maximum number of prisoners held by the British at any one time was about 5500.

Both the colonists and the British held prisoners in buildings, stockades, or hastily erected prisons—wherever the fighting happened to be. Most prisons were abandoned as the fighting moved from place to place. Many prisoners of the British were either paroled if they promised not to rejoin the army or exchanged for British prisoners. Some captured British officers were even allowed to stay in colonists' homes!

It soon became apparent to both sides that they were not prepared for the large number of prisoners captured during the first-year hostilities. Accordingly, GEN Sir William Howe appointed Joshua Loring as the first Commanding General of Prisons, establishing the colonists' ration as two-thirds that of the British. Although Loring did not intentionally abuse or neglect his charges, they were subjected to corruption by prison officials, poor quality food, and the low state of medical care of the time. Further distress was endured when American POWs were crammed into suffocating warehouses.

Finally, British leaders consented to parole American officers who agreed to live in Loyalist homes around New York City. This, plus the use of British ships—not sturdy or swift enough for combat—as prisons, somewhat eased the crowding. Still, these floating penitentiaries were miserable places where men lived in dank, dark cells in which disease spread rapidly. It is estimated that 700 colonials died on these ships.

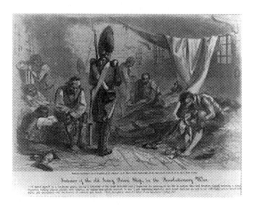

Colonial POWs aboard British prison ship
"HMS *Jersey*." Creative Commons.

By 1780, an estimated 5300 American prisoners were held on ships and in Great Britain, including seamen from allied nations such as France, as well as colonial crews caught in non-American waters. Benjamin Franklin, then serving as a diplomat in Paris, was able to deliver aid to POWs held in England through his connections in Parliament. He also requested additional funds from Congress, which were limited. Even here, corruption reigned, and guards still served maggoty beef and watered-down beer.

Escape was difficult because most prisoners lacked the physical strength and courage to attempt it. Furthermore, recapture involved severe punishment—even being placed in irons. Some prisoners secured their release by enlisting in the British army or navy—recruiters were not hard to reach. Some inmates mistakenly believed that conditions were intentional. Parole, of course, was another means of gaining freedom but, again, infraction of the privilege was subject to severe punishment. Isaac Hayne, a militia colonel from South Carolina, was executed for violating parole. (GEN Ethan Allen, leader of the Green Mountain Boys, was probably the best-known parolee.) Even GEN Washington was unsuccessful in persuading the British to establish formal exchange policies. However, after GEN Burgoyne surrendered several thousand prisoners at Saratoga in 1777, the colonists gained some leverage in exchange discussions. In the years following, Britain came to agree to exchange several thousand prisoners, including Ethan Allen. By July 1783, all but a few Hessians had been released.[4]

WAR OF 1812

Compared with the Revolutionary War, the War of 1812 generally witnessed humane treatment of POWs of both sides. This conflict was initiated by President James Madison against Great Britain as a result of sanctions brought by Britain and France during the Napoleonic Wars and in outrage over Britain's impressment of American seamen. After the British victory at Detroit in August 1812, resolution of remaining conflicts followed a similar pattern: Members of volunteer units and militia who surrendered were normally dismissed after having promised that they would not serve again, while regular troops were held for longer periods. Officers were usually paroled with freedom of movement within a particular town or area, but enlisted men were often incarcerated for years before they could be exchanged for prisoners from the other side.[5]

The opposing factions entered into several conventions, the first signed at Halifax, Nova Scotia, in November 1812. Upon the consent of both parties, an exchange of lists would occur and POWs and soldiers on parole behind enemy lines on both sides would be free to return to their countries. The agreement even specified the comparative value of individuals involved: one sergeant was the equivalent of two privates; a colonel equaled two privates; a brigadier general was worth 30 privates.

The following year, a second negotiation declared that captives were to be treated with "humanity, comformable to the usage and practice of the most civilized nations during the war," and corporal punishment was prohibited. Unfortunately, Britain failed to ratify the agreement, presumably disagreeing with the type of food required by the Americans and their insistence on the parole of maritime captives. Nevertheless, the main principles of both conventions were generally adhered to.

Yet, there were two incidents that brought out the retaliatory attitudes of both sides. In the first, the British threatened to prosecute 23 American soldiers for treason on the grounds that they were British subjects, despite naturalization. The Americans retaliated by threatening to execute double the number of British POWs. The ante kept rising until cooler heads prevailed and a prisoner exchange was arranged.

The other incident occurred in January 1813 in present-day Michigan when the British defeated an American army at River Raisin. Most of the colonists were marched back to British territory but 80 were left behind because they were unable to walk. Immediately the unprotected prisoners were set upon by a gang of native warriors attached to the enemy forces, killing 30 of them, torturing a few others, and holding the rest for ransom.[6]

Approximately 25,000 Americans—mostly seamen— were imprisoned by the British over the course of the war, yet only 275 died, mostly from pneumonia and smallpox. With the signing of the Treaty of Ghent on December 24, 1814, all territorial conquests of both sides were returned, heralding two centuries of peace between the two nations. For Native Americans who allied with the British, however, the war had devastated their physical land and political autonomy and destroyed their power to block American expansion into the Northwest.[7]

MEXICAN-AMERICAN WAR

When Mexico refused diplomatic efforts by the United States to purchase the territories of New Mexico and California, war fever seized the territories, intensified by recent memories of the Mexican annihilation of American prisoners at the Alamo in 1836, as well as other instances of imprisonment of Americans in Mexican territories. The immediate cause of the war was a border dispute arising out of the 1845 US annexation of Texas. War with Mexico was supported by imperialists and proponents of slavery.

Each battle saw the capture of several thousand Mexican prisoners, including priests acting as guerrillas directing attacks against Americans. US troops usually exchanged or paroled prisoners to avoid the cost of sheltering and supplying them. However, some officers refused parole, forcing the US government to transfer them to the United States at considerable expense.

The number of Americans imprisoned by the Mexicans is not well documented, but it is known that the prisoners were used for labor. They were also paraded through towns to boost public support for the war. Each side claimed that the other was cruel while depicting their own guards as humane. The Burlington (Iowa) *Hawk-Eye* reported that when MAJ Frederick D. Mills tried to surrender, "the Mexicans basely fell upon him and lanced him to death." Soldiers of both sides willingly accepted the spoils of war. One US soldier, after a successful attack on Chapultepec Castle, was permitted to choose a horse that had belonged to an imprisoned Mexican officer.

Some deserters from the American army, who had been enticed by offers of money, property, or rank, were court-martialed when recaptured and literally drummed out of the service to the tune of "The Rogue's March." The editor of the *American Star* called them "apostasized and toad-spotted traitors" for whom "feelings of loathing and disgust take possession of us . . ."[8]

In a discussion of prisoner exchange near the war's end, Archbishop Manuel of Mexico City offered to administer an oath to 800 Mexican POWs that they would honor their parole on pain of execution if caught. MG Winfield Scott answered that his past requests for the exchange of several Americans had been ignored. He finally relented after the archbishop agreed to Scott's demand that parolees who reenlisted would be executed if caught. It was so carried out.

The February 1848 Treaty of Guadalupe Hidalgo revealed that many Mexicans had been captured by Native American warriors, especially Comanches. Accordingly, one of the treaty's provisions was that "the government of the United States will exact the release of such captives and cause them to be restored to their country." At the Citadel

(Monterey, Calif), MG William O. Butler, Scott's successor, ordered the buttons of American deserters to be removed and to set the deserters free. However, to some, "freedom" meant begging on the streets to survive.[9]

THE CIVIL WAR

The War Between the States produced some of the most notorious instances of prisoner abuse in American history. For the first 2 years of the war, as a result of the policy of early prisoner exchange and parole, the POW problems were manageable. However, because of the Union's reluctance to deal with their Confederate counterparts for fear of appearing to recognize the South as a legitimate government, in July 1862 the Dix-Hill cartel regulating prisoner exchange was inaugurated.

Unfortunately, the cartel broke down in mid-1863 due to issues relating to race, ie, the North's growing insistence on emancipation (culminating in the Emancipation Proclamation) and its decision to raise black regiments. The South announced a policy of executing white officers leading black troops and treating captured African American soldiers as rebellious slaves even though they were originally free. It was suspected that black soldiers died in numbers and under circumstances that they feared dire consequences if captured much more than did their white counterparts.

With the tens of thousands of prisoners taken in 1863 and '64, the suspension of the cartel overburdened the inadequately prepared prison systems of both sides. Union troops were especially hard-hit by the suspension, suffering from the consequences of the ill-planned, ill-run, and ill-supplied Southern prison camps. The largest and most notorious of these was at Andersonville, Georgia. Officially known as Camp Sumter, it was built to enable the South to relocate the prisoners housed in and around Richmond to a more secure location and one where more food supplies were available. More than 45,000 Union soldiers were housed here during the 14 months of its existence.

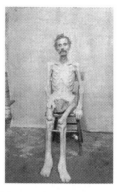

Union Army soldier on his release from Andersonville prison in May 1865. Public Domain.

"Housed" is hardly the appropriate term—the prisoners were simply herded into an open stockade and left to fend for themselves. There were neither barracks nor a hospital. A small stream that cut across the yard served as the prisoners' sole source of water, but it soon became polluted by the human waste and refuse that was collected. Smallpox, typhoid, diarrhea, dysentery, scurvy, and pneumonia were rife. Of these 45,000 POWs, almost one-third died from malnutrition, poor sanitation, or exposure.

These conditions were aggravated by the fact that the facility was less than half completed when the first captives arrived in February 1864. By the end of June, 26,000 men had been confined in a 26 ½-acre area originally intended for only 10,000. By August, the number had swelled to 33,000. Because of the deteriorating economic conditions and the poor transportation system, the Confederate government was unable to adequately house, feed, clothe, or provide medical care for their captives or adequately address the army's desperate need for food and supplies.

The April 1864 exchange of the sickest prisoners revealed the suffering the Union troops had undergone, leading many Northerners to accuse the Confederacy of deliberately starving Union POWs. The following month, Secretary of War Edwin Stanton retaliated by cutting the rations of Confederate prisoners. The popular ballad, "Tramp! Tramp! Tramp! The Boys Are Marching," typified the unforgiving and ultrapatriotic mood of most Northerners. Many white Southerners accused GEN Grant of suspending prisoner exchanges to aggravate the severe manpower problems of the South.

When GEN William T. Sherman's Union forces occupied nearby Atlanta in September 1864, Confederate officials moved most of the prisoners to other camps on Georgia's coast and in South Carolina, reducing Andersonville's population. Along with the diminishing occupancy, however, sanitary conditions and medical care further deteriorated. The resumption of prisoner exchanges and transfer of inmates to other facilities brought some relief, but it was too late to save the almost 13,000 lives that had been lost in Andersonville's killing fields.

When a large hospital was finally erected in April 1865, the surgeons were soon overwhelmed. Most of the ill died in the dirt where they collapsed. More than 1500 died in the first 3 months. The stockade commander, CPT Henry Wirz, repeatedly requested sufficient rations, but a combination of bureaucratic quarreling, scarcity, and officials' naïveté ensured that the prisoners were doomed to slow starvation.

The Confederates, in critical military straits by January 1865—and possibly thinking of the desperate measure of recruiting African Americans into their own forces—agreed to a rapid prisoner exchange, including black Union soldiers. After the major Northern victories of April 1865, Southern troops, rather than being taken into captivity, were allowed to return home on parole. The remaining prisoners on both sides were also released.

When the war ended in April 1865, the final casualty of the prison at Fort Sumter was ironically the camp's commandant, Henry Wirz, who was charged, along with certain Confederate officials, for conspiring to "impair and injure the health and destroy the lives . . . of Federal prisoners" and "murder in violation of the laws of war." Such a conspiracy had never existed but someone had to be the scapegoat—such was the anger and indignation of the North over conditions at Andersonville. After a carefully scripted trial, Wirz was found guilty of the atrocities and hung on November 10, 1865, the only person executed for war crimes during the Civil War.

Of the 195,000 Union soldiers who died in the Civil War, over 15% died while prisoners; of the 215,000 Confederate dead, almost 12% died in captivity, making the Civil War America's bloodiest conflict. Almost as many men died in captivity during the Civil War as were killed in the entire Vietnam War.[10]

SPANISH-AMERICAN WAR

The War with Spain brings to mind the sinking of the battleship *Maine* and the exploits of Theodore (Teddy)

Roosevelt and his Rough Riders, who assisted in the capture of the city of Santiago de Cuba in July 1898.

Because the United States abided by the terms of the 1864 Geneva Convention, it was obliged to protect its Spanish prisoners from its Cuban and Filipino allies. All in all, the treatment of its 39,000 Spanish prisoners was humane. After they surrendered their weapons, the Spanish prisoners were held with only minimal restrictions, even fraternizing with their American captors. In contrast, Spain held only a few Americans.

After the Battle of Santiago Bay, the entire Spanish fleet consisted of only 1774 prisoners. These were distributed between Norfolk, Virginia; Fort McPherson, Georgia; Seavey Island, New Hampshire; and the US Naval Academy at Annapolis, Maryland, where the best treatment was found. Officers there who signed a parole were permitted liberty in town.

The Spanish navy's most noteworthy prisoner, Admiral (ADM) Pascual Cervera y Popete, refused to sign a parole because he asserted that it was prohibited by Spanish law; as a result, he was granted liberty based on his word as a gentleman. To avoid his being insulted by being a captive of a lower-ranking officer, the academy's superintendent was replaced with Rear Admiral (RDML) Frederick McNair, who provided the Spaniard and his son with a house on the academy's campus and servants. He was also allowed to socialize with local Annapolis residents at parties and church services.

To avoid the unwanted burden of protecting the 13,000 Spanish prisoners remaining in the Philippines—vulnerable to the brutal attacks of rebel forces of Emelio Aguinaldo's rebel forces—the United States quickly agreed to pay their transportation back to Spain. As a result of their victory over Spain, the United States emerged as a world power and gained possession of Guam, Puerto Rico, and the Philippines.[11]

WORLD WAR I

The Great War was truly a war of the world, involving as it did 32 countries. The Allies, or Entente Powers, consisting of France, the United Kingdom, the United States, Russia, Japan, and Italy, were opposed by the Central Powers— Germany, Austria-Hungary, the Ottoman Empire, and Bulgaria. Each side was joined by numerous allies. Because of the widespread battlefields, it is convenient to divide our discussion into four main fronts: Eastern, Middle Eastern, Ottoman Empire, and Western.

Eastern (Russian) Front. The chief belligerent powers on the Eastern Front were Russia, on the Allied side, and Germany and Austria-Hungary of the Central Powers. The most notable feature of the Eastern Front was the huge numbers of prisoners taken by both sides. During the 3 ½ years of hostilities, 5 million soldiers were taken captive on the Eastern Front, with Russia capturing the most (about 2.27 million). At the Battle of Lutsk (Ukraine) alone in June 1916, the Austro-Hungarian army lost 240,000 captives.

All major Eastern Front participants had signed the Hague conventions of 1899 and 1907, so they were obliged to treat their POWs in a "humane" manner and, in general, they did. Nonetheless, their complete lack of preparedness to feed, clothe, and house the huge numbers of captives meant that actual conditions in the camps—especially the Russian camps— quickly became substandard, particularly during the first two years of the war, when outbreaks of typhus, typhoid fever, and dysentery were reported on both sides.

With the construction of more permanent camps and usage of POW labor (providing supplemental income), prisoners' living conditions began to improve. The Bolshevik Revolution of March 1917 brought in a less restrictive regime. However, the political chaos brought about by the ensuing civil war disrupted official policies and left the prisoners at the mercy of local commandants.

POW commissioned officers, in contrast to rank-and-file prisoners, were treated as gentlemen. Consequently, they received a monthly salary, better quarters, exemption from labor, and permission to present theatrical productions, organize self-improvement classes, and make purchases outside camp. Toward the end of the war, however, inflationary pressures and scarcity of food, especially in the German-speaking countries, reduced the gap between their living conditions and those of the enlisted personnel.

Not long after an aborted peace talk between Russia and Germany in December 1917, Vladimir Lenin, fearing an advance of German troops on St Petersburg, signed the Treaty of Brest-Litovsk (Poland) on March 3, 1918, effectively eliminating Russia from the war 8 months before what was to be the main armistice.

Unfortunately, as a result of a delay in negotiations for the duration of the Russian Civil War (1918-20), some 500,000 Central Powers POWs were trapped in Siberia and central Asia—and some 200,000 Russian prisoners were likewise prevented from returning home. The last prisoners were not released until the spring of 1922.[12]

Middle Eastern—Ottoman Empire. Those Allied forces—mostly British and Indian—who fell into Turkish hands suffered almost unequaled brutality. Nearly 13,000

British and Indian prisoners were taken by the Turks in the April 1915 defeat at Kut-al-Amara. Although the officers, including members of the Royal Flying Corps, were treated in an acceptable— though Spartan—manner, the rank-and-file troops suffered atrocious treatment and died by the thousands.

Their ordeal began on the march from Kut to Baghdad when a combination of wounds, disease, exhaustion, and lack of food and water decimated their ranks. By the time the survivors had reached Ras al Ain, over 3000 of them had died. Those remaining were put to work on the Baghdad Railway. Only through considerable effort were neutral observers—notably American diplomatic officials—allowed to administer aid to the prisoners. By then it was too late for many: 70% of the British POWs and 27% of the Indians had died. Despite the deplorable conditions endured by the prisoners, it must be remembered that overcrowding, poor rations, vermin infestation, and primitive living quarters were typical of the Turkish soldiers' own lot.[13]

In contrast to the limited numbers of Entente captives taken, the prisoner count of Ottomans in World War I was in the hundreds of thousands, estimated at 250,000. The largest group of these, close to 150,000, had been captured by the British, the next largest by the Russians, who held between 61,000 and 90,000, while the French had at most 2000.

The Russian Empire was seriously unprepared to handle the large numbers of prisoners it had captured, As a result, captives of the Central Powers captives were housed in makeshift, overcrowded, and unsanitary facilities, resulting in outbreaks of typhus and other diseases. Some Turkish prisoners froze to death en route to prison camps because of Russian indifference and neglect. Most, with the exception of officers, were interned in Siberia employed in Russian industry where conditions were worse than in European Russia. Some 25% of Ottoman prisoners held by the Russians died in captivity.

Ottomans captured in Egypt encountered a less onerous lifestyle than did their compatriots in Russia because of the more moderate, better hygienic conditions, and newly constructed camps. Little is known about the 18,000 Ottoman POWs held in India and Burma. Prisoners in Britain's far-flung prison camps tried to alleviate their boredom and become more productive by organizing courses and workshops to learn foreign languages and new skills or to simply learn to read and write.

Adding to the usual diseases and other trials imposed on Turkish POWs of the Middle East–Ottoman front was the fact that 10% were blind in one or both eyes on repatriation, most likely as a result of trachoma, an infectious eye disease prevalent in that area.[13]

Western Front*.* Hostilities on the Western Front were set apart by the facts of mechanization, trench warfare, and mostly stagnant battlefields. However, large groups of prisoners were taken by both sides during the open-warfare phases of 1914 and 1918. During the Entente spring offensive of 1918, around 100,000 British soldiers were taken prisoner. The war's end found 6577 British officers and 161,026 enlisted men in German camps. About 328,000 German POWs had been captured by the British and 400,000 by the French, who also held a number of Turkish and Bulgarian prisoners on the island of Corsica.

Out of some 65,000 Austro-Hungarian prisoners captured by Serbia, only about 20,000 remained by the time they reached camps in France due to disease, wounds, and accidents. Other special groups, such as Danes from

Schleswig, Franco-Germans from Alsace-Lorraine, Bulgarians, and a number of Austro-Hungarians were viewed sympathetically by the French and were culled out for favored prisoner status.

The best conditions for POWs were found in Britain and in France by the American Expeditionary Force after entering the fray in April 1917. Slightly less favorable conditions prevailed in the French-run camps, while by far the worst circumstances were found in the German work camps. As was typical, officers thrived somewhat better. Even US camps were initially overcrowded and had inadequate facilities.

Initially the French extended parole to officer prisoners until they learned that the Germans were not doing so to their French POWs. Likewise, the French abided by the Hague Convention, not forcing prisoners to work in war-related industries, whereas not so the German captors. Accordingly, these practices were stopped, and the French kept the German POWs working on war damage almost 2 years beyond the armistice as a form of retribution. Even so, considering conditions in postwar Germany, the POWs may have been better off staying in France.

The plight of those captured by the Germans depended to a great extent on where they ended up. Those lucky enough to be assigned to agricultural camps had relatively pleasant work and the possibility of obtaining extra food. Those sent to industrial plants managed by sensible businessmen who understood that contented workers were the most efficient fared almost as well. But many more were forced to work in dangerous conditions under the supervision of brutal overseers. Minor cuts usually went untreated, with blood poisoning often the outcome. Arms and legs caught in machinery produced frightful results. Prisoners working in the salt mines developed painful sores on their arms and legs. POWs found to be working too slowly were beaten. Many former prisoners found that the aftereffects of these abuses left lifelong physical and emotional scars.

Compared with World War II, escape was less dangerous and had a higher chance of success because (1) anti-escape techniques were more primitive, (2) the police in the larger community were less vigilant, and (3) if recaptured, they generally received lighter punishments. Escapees able to reach the German border found neutral havens in The Netherlands and Switzerland. Germans and others able to escape British prison camps latched onto the Dutch ships that frequented British ports.

Prisoners who were seriously sick or wounded, over a certain age, or who had spent over 18 months in captivity were either released to their own countries or allowed to sit out the war in neutral Holland, Sweden, or Switzerland, according to agreements made by belligerents on the Western Front. To many of the 145,000 POWs of both sides, this meant the difference between life and death.

The armistice of November 11, 1918, did not spell freedom for many captives. POWs in France and Britain were kept working as a form of punishment; a large segment of the Allied population thought that the Germans should clean up the damage caused by the war. In Germany, central authority had largely broken down, leaving the prisoners at the mercy of local authorities. A number of the guards had simply deserted and many of the British prisoners had to make their way out of Germany on their own. Those in the east found this extremely difficult: men released from the Stralsund camp on the Baltic coast had to charter a special train to transport them to Denmark.[14] And, in many ways, because of the harsh penalties imposed on Germany by the Treaty of Versailles, all the bloodshed and misery brought about by 3 ½ years of war only set the stage for another war 21 years later.

REFERENCES FOR CHAPTER V

1   The fate of prisoners of war. *The Week*. 2007. Available at: https://
    theweek.com/articles/528999/fate-prisoners-war. Accessed July 5,
    2018.

2   Dunant H. *A Memory of Solferino*. 2019. Available at: https://
    en.wikipedia.org/wiki/A_Memory_of_Solferino.   Accessed
    October 22, 2019.

3   Geneva Conventions. Available at: https://en.wikipedia.org/wiki/
    Geneva_Conventions. Accessed May 12, 2019.

4   Prisoners of war in the American Revolutionary War. Available
    at: https://en.wikipedia.org/wiki/Prisoners_of_war_in_the_
    American_ Revolutionary_War. Accessed February 2, 2019.

5   War of 1812. Available at: https://en.wikipedia.org/wiki/War_of_
    1812. Accessed December 21, 2019.

6   River Raisin—Battles of Frenchtown. Available at: https://www.
    battlefields.org/learn/war-1812/battles/river-raisin.   Accessed
    December 21, 2019.

7   Sheppard G. War of 1812 (1812-1815). In Vance JF, Ed. *Encyclopedia
    of Prisoners of War and Internment*. Santa Barbara, Calif: ABC-
    CLIO; 2000: 312-315.

8   Shafer ED. Mexican-American War (1846-1848). In Vance,
    186-187.

9   Gardner DG. United States Civil War (1861-1865). In Vance, 9,
    10, 297-299.

10 Spanish-American War. Available at: https://en.wikipedia.org/
    wiki/Spanish%E2%80%93American_War. Accessed March 17,
    2019.

11 Rachamimov A. World War I—Eastern Front. In Vance, 321-323.

12 Vance JF. World War I—Middle East. In Vance, 324-325.

13 Yanikdag Y. World War I—Ottoman Empire. In Vance, 325-326.

14 Vance JF. World War I—Western Front. In Vance, 326-329.

VI

POWS OF US WARS, WWII TO GULF WAR

WORLD WAR I I

The following section, discussing the primary fronts, is divided into three parts: Western Europe, the Eastern Front, and the Far East.

Western Europe. It was as if the world's inhabitants had been asked to come up with living quarters for a country the size of The Netherlands or a city the size of New York and its environs. That is about the number of prisoners captured in the 5 ½-year period of World War II needing to be housed, fed, and medically cared for. This figure includes between 8 ½ and 9 million Allied POWs (6 million of whom were Soviets) and 8 ¼ million Germans and Italians, and does not, of course, include the millions involved in the other theaters of war.

The conditions provided by the belligerents of the Second World War fell far short of the provisions of the 1929 Convention Relative to the Treatment of Prisoners of War, especially for those prisoners whose countries had been overrun by the Germans. The most notable consequence was the use of French and Belgian POWs in the German munitions industry. However, the Allies had one bargaining chip: the large number of German prisoners under their control and the threat of reprisal thus afforded.

Another prisoner abuse was the shackling of British and Canadian troops for a year after the Germans had accused the Allies of binding the hands of the German captives during the raid on Dieppe in 1942. The Germans also reduced the rations of US and British POWs in accordance with the bounty of foodstuffs given the prisoners by the Red Cross, thus forcing the home countries to subsidize German obligations under the Hague Convention. After the United States entered the war, both sides made good use of the Swiss government as the official protecting power, allowing their representatives as well as the International Committee of the Red Cross (ICRC) unlimited access in inspecting the camps. Of course, it was only human nature for the camp officials to let the visitors see only what they wanted them to see.

Early in the war, both sides made accusations of mass killings, including those made by units of the Waffen-SS. Hitler's Commando Order of October 1942 led to the killing of small groups of Allied commandos, which became the basis for accusations of war crimes at the postwar Nuremberg Trials. For their part, the German government accused the Brits of killing their captives during the Greek campaign. While many of these accusations were unfounded, it is probable that some excesses were committed by both sides that went unreported and were, therefore, unpunished. Although some have questioned the Allies' treatment of German prisoners immediately after the Armistice, there is no doubt that, in general, their treatment was far superior to that of the German treatment of American and British POWs.[1]

Eastern Front. Approximately 3 million German prisoners of war were captured by the Soviet Union during World War II, most of them during the great advances of the Red Army in the last year of the war. These POWs were employed as forced labor in the Soviet wartime economy and in the postwar reconstruction. By 1950 almost all surviving POWs had been released, with the last prisoner returning from the USSR in 1956. According to Soviet records, 381,067 German *Wehrmacht* POWs died in NKVD (roughly, the secret police) camps (356,700 German nationals and 24,367 from other nations). It is estimated that one million died in Soviet custody. In the first months of Operation Barbarossa, few Germans were captured by Soviet forces.

By early 1942, after the Battle of Moscow and the retreat of the German forces, the number of prisoners in the Soviet prisoner of war camps rose to 120,000. When the German 6th Army surrendered after the Battle of Stalingrad in early 1943, 91,000 of the survivors became prisoners of war, raising the total to 211,000. Weakened by disease, starvation, and lack of medical care during the encirclement, many died of wounds, disease (particularly typhus), malnutrition, and maltreatment in the months following their capture at Stalingrad: only approximately 6000 lived to be repatriated after the war. As the desperate economic situation in the Soviet Union eased in 1943, the mortality rate in the POW camps sank dramatically. At the same time, POWs became an important source of labor for the manpower-deprived Soviet economy. As a result of Operation Bagration and the collapse on the southern part of the Eastern front in the second half of 1944, the number of German POWs nearly doubled. In the first months of 1945, the Red Army advanced to the Oder River and on the Balkans. Again the number of POWs rose–to 2 million by April 1945.

A total of 2.8 million German *Wehrmacht* personnel were held as POWs by the Soviet Union at the end of the war, according to Soviet records. With the creation of a pro-Soviet German state in the Soviet occupation zone of Germany—the German Democratic Republic—in October 1949, all but 85,000 POWs had been released and repatriated. Most of those still held had been convicted of war crimes and had been sentenced to lengthy terms, usually 25 years in forced labor camps. It was not until 1956, after the intervention of West German Chancellor Konrad Adenauer in Moscow, that the last of these "war convicts" were repatriated.

Nazi Germany engaged in a policy of deliberate maltreatment of Soviet POWs, in contrast to their treatment of British and American POWs. Hitler had instructed his troops, for this campaign, to ignore the code of military honor. "The Communist is from first to last no comrade. It is a war of extermination."[2]

This resulted in some 3.3 to 3.5 million deaths. Many were executed arbitrarily in the field by the German forces or handed over to the SS to be shot, under the Commissar Order, which was a written order given by the German High Command on 6 June 1941, prior to the beginning of the German invasion of the Soviet Union. The Order demanded that any Soviet political commissar identified among captured troops be shot immediately. Those prisoners who could be identified as "thoroughly bolshevized or as active representatives of the Bolshevist ideology" were also to be executed. Most, however, died during the death marches from the front lines or under inhumane conditions in German prisoner-of-war camps and concentration camps.

It has been estimated that at least 3.3 million of the 5.7 million Soviet POWs died in Nazi custody. This figure represents a total of 57% of all Soviet POWs and may be contrasted with the deaths of 8300 out of 231,000 British and U.S. prisoners, or 3.6%. About 5% of the Soviet prisoners who died were Jews. The largest number of deaths took place between June 1941 and January 1942, when the Germans killed an estimated 2.8 million Soviet POWs primarily through deliberate starvation, exposure, and summary execution.

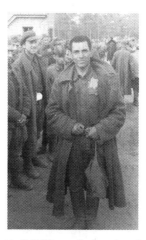

Jewish-Soviet POWs marked with yellow badges,
August 1941. Creative Commons.

By September 1941, the mortality rate among Soviet POWs was about 1% per day. According to the United States Holocaust Memorial Museum, by the winter of 1941, "starvation and disease resulted in mass death of unimaginable proportions." This deliberate starvation, despite the availability of adequate food supplies, led many desperate prisoners to resort to acts of cannibalism. For the

Germans, Soviet POWs were expendable: They consumed calories needed by others and, unlike Western POWs, were considered to be subhuman.

In the summer and autumn of 1941, vast numbers of Soviet prisoners were captured in about a dozen large encirclements. As a result of their rapid advance into the Soviet Union and an anticipated quick victory, the Germans did not want to ship these prisoners to Germany. Under the administration of the *Wehrmacht*, the prisoners were processed, guarded, forced-marched, or transported in open rail cars to locations mostly in the occupied Soviet Union, Germany, and occupied Poland. Much like comparable events, such as the Pacific War's Bataan Death March in 1942, the treatment of prisoners was brutal, with little in the way of supporting logistics.

Soviet prisoners of war were stripped of their supplies and clothing by poorly-equipped German troops when the cold weather set in, resulting in death for many of the prisoners. Most of the camps for Soviet POWs were simply open areas fenced off with barbed wire and watchtowers with no inmate housing. These meager conditions forced the crowded prisoners to live in holes they had dug for themselves, exposed to the elements. Beatings and other abuse by the guards were common, and prisoners were malnourished, often consuming only a few hundred calories or less per day. Medical treatment was nonexistent and an International Red Cross offer of assistance in 1941 was rejected by Hitler.

Some of the Soviet POWs were also made subjects of experimentation. In one such case, Dr. Heinrich Berning of Hamburg University starved prisoners to death as "famine experiments." In another instance, a group of prisoners at Zhitomir were shot using dum-dum bullets (bullets designed to expand on impact). Although Allied regulars kept by Germany were usually treated in accordance with the 1929 Geneva Convention on Prisoners of War, conditions for the Soviets were far worse.[3]

Far East. Approximately 320,000 Allied soldiers were captured by Japan during World War II. Of these, 140,000 were European and North Americans, whereas 180,000 were Asians. Although most nonwhites were released within a few months of capture, most whites were held until the end of the war in 1945. Of prisoners in captivity, 8288 (35.6%) Americans died. Combining prisoners of all nationalities, 37,800 men (26.9%) perished. In a monumental display of opportunism, Russia entered the war against Japan after the atomic bomb had been dropped and took (so they claimed) 594,000 Japanese soldiers captive (Japanese scholars put the figure at 850,000), shipping them to Siberia, where they remained for several years.

Since Japan's military law forbids surrender, the Allies took far fewer prisoners than did the Russians. For example, out of 30,000 original Japanese troops, only 1400 survived to break out of Allied encirclement. At Iwo Jima, only 216 remained of the original 21,000 in the main garrison. Some historians attribute this to more than Japanese law: Once Allied troops learned of Japanese atrocities, they simply stopped taking prisoners.

Allied personnel received far better treatment from the Germans than they did from the Japanese: While only about 4% of Allied troops died in German hands, approximately 27% perished in Japanese captivity. Japanese POWs in American, British, Australian, and New Zealand were, in general, humanely—though frugally—treated. Although the Japanese had signed the Hague Convention of 1907, their promise, for the most part, had not been kept. Early on, Japanese Prime Minister Hideki Tojo issued orders that POWs were to work for their keep. In violation of international law, they were regularly used in war-related industries, such as building bridges and forts and digging trenches. For this, they were fed a starvation diet. Once their uniforms wore out, no replacements were provided. Some prison guards answered requests for water with beatings or rifle butts.

Prisoners who were seen as not useful, eg, physically weak or rebellious, were often killed. Other atrocities included filling a prisoner's nose with water while guards tied them with barbed wire and stood on their recumbent bodies. Or the guards tied them by their thumbs to a tree limb so that their feet barely touched the ground and then left them there for two days without food or water. At the end of the war, when the camp inmates were released, many had lost body parts or were so starved that they resembled walking skeletons. Traumatized prisoners suffered mental illnesses that persisted for decades afterward.[4]

In some camps, prisoners were fattened up to be killed and eaten. At great risk, artist-prisoners recorded life in the camp using human hair for brushes, plant juice or blood for paint, and toilet paper as the "canvas." Some of these drawings were used as evidence in the trials of Japanese war criminals. To add to their misery, the Red Cross was unable to drop parcels from the air because the camps were too well defended to fly over. When prisoners were transported, they were herded along in death marches, crowded into unendurably hot boxcars, or packed for days into the sweltering holds of "death ships" with little or no room to move and nowhere to perform bodily functions. As one writer has put it, prisoners of the Japanese endured "hell on earth: aging faster, dying sooner."[5]

Norman Wahl, DDS, MS, MA

GERMAN POWS IN THE UNITED STATES

It is not widely remembered that 425,000 German prisoners of war were held in 700 camps in the United States during and after World War II. Almost all German-speaking Americans were overseas involved in combat efforts and the American government feared the presence of Germans on US soil would create a security problem and raise fear among civilians.

Despite many rumors about how the Allies treated their prisoners, some Germans were pleased to be captured by the British or Americans— while fear of being captured by the Soviets was widespread. For prisoners held by Americans, good treatment began with the substantial meals served aboard the troopships transporting them to America, even though they risked being torpedoed by their own submarines. Upon arriving in the United States, the POWs were amazed by the comfort of the Pullman cars that carried them to their camps, as did the country's vast size and undamaged property. The Geneva Convention of 1929 required the United States to provide living quarters comparable to its own military, which meant 40 square feet per individual for enlisted men and 120 square feet for officers. The 40 generals and three admirals in custody were sent to Camp Shelby, Mississippi, where each had his own bungalow with a garden.

As millions of soldiers were overseas, the resulting shortage of labor eventually meant that German POWs worked toward the Allied war effort by being assigned to canneries, mills, and farms that were deemed a minimal security risk. Prisoners could not be used in work directly related to the war effort or in dangerous conditions. The minimum pay for soldiers was 80 cents a day, roughly equivalent to the pay of an American private. While prisoners on average worked more slowly and produced less than civilians, their work was also more reliable and of higher quality. They were paid in scrip, because all hard currency had been confiscated along with personal possessions, as money could be used in escape attempts.[6]

While most US citizens living near camps accepted the prisoners' presence, the government received hundreds of letters each week protesting their treatment, many demanding that the POWs be immediately killed. The government had difficulty in persuading the public that treating the prisoners according to the Geneva Convention made it more likely that Germany would treat American prisoners well. Given the wartime labor shortage, however, especially in agriculture, many valued their contribution; as late as February 1945, politicians in rural states were asking the government for 100,000 more prisoners to work on farms.

Because there was insufficient manpower to provide American guards, especially German speakers, emphasis was placed mostly on supervising the German officers and NCOs who, in turn, maintained strict discipline among the enlisted men. They awakened their own men, marched them to meals, and prepared them for work. Prisoners had friendly interaction with local civilians and sometimes were allowed outside the camp on the honor system without guards (African American guards noted that prisoners could visit segregated restaurants that they themselves could not). Sometimes, unauthorized fraternization between American women and German prisoners occurred. Several camps held social receptions with local American women, and some Germans met their future wives this way.

The prisoners were provided with writing materials, art supplies, woodworking tools, and musical instruments, and were allowed regular correspondence with family in Germany. General officers received wine with their meals, and all prisoners received the same rations as American soldiers, as required by the Geneva Convention. Prisoners held frequent musical and theatrical performances attended by hundreds or thousands. Movies were shown as often as four nights a week. After the liberation of the Nazi concentration camps in Germany, films of the Holocaust atrocities were shown to the prisoners, engendering shock, anger, and disbelief. After compulsory viewing of one atrocity film, 1000 prisoners at Camp Butner dramatically burned their German uniforms. A few prisoners even volunteered to fight in the war against Japan.

Every camp published its own newspaper, and camp authorities recognized the periodicals' value as indicators of prisoners' views. Even as Germany's defeat neared in early 1945, 8 of 20 camp newspapers still advocated Nazi ideology. Some prisoners took correspondence courses through universities—German universities also accepted their credits after they returned home.[5]

Despite efforts to isolate devoted Nazis and other fanatics, some were able to lead work stoppages, intimidate other prisoners, and hold secret kangaroo courts for those accused of disloyalty. Those convicted were sometimes attacked or killed. Most prisoner "suicides" were likely murders. Many prisoners remained loyal to their political beliefs and up to the last minute expected a German victory. They secretly celebrated Hitler's birthday and other Nazi holidays and resented supervision by American Jewish officers. As for escape, the likelihood of returning to their forces overseas was very remote: less than 1% of POWs in America attempted it.

Korean War. On June 25, 1950, the Communist North Korean People's Army, without warning, attacked the Free Republic of South Korea. During the ensuing 3 years of warfare, the North Koreans committed a series of war crimes against American and United Nations personnel that constituted one of the most atrocious and barbaric epochs of recorded history.

The treatment of prisoners of war and their repatriation was a complicated issue of the involvement of 16 members of the United Nations. The North Koreans were joined by the Chinese Peoples' Volunteer Forces, attempts at brainwashing were widespread, and the South Koreans were treated differently than other UN members. At the time of the Armistice, there were 13,803 United Nations Command (UNC) POWs (including 3746 Americans) and 105,097 communist prisoners, including 21,721 Chinese. MG William F. Dean was the highest-ranking UNC officer captured by the North Koreans.

Nominally, both the Communist and United Nations forces were committed to the terms of the 1949 Third Geneva Convention regarding the treatment of POWs. Both sides claimed exceptions, however, and the negotiations regarding POWs were contentious and difficult. Citing the terms of the 1949 Geneva Convention, the Chinese and North Koreans demanded total repatriation of their POWs, whereas the UNC insisted on "voluntary repatriation" based on humanitarian issues. Two-thirds of the Chinese refused to be repatriated because they feared being persecuted, as were the Russians who were returned to the Soviet Union after World War II (only 10% of the North Koreans declined repatriation). Most of the 7017 Chinese POWs who returned to mainland China were purged, and many were expelled from the Communist party, deprived of employment opportunities, forced to divorce, or sent to hard labor.[7]

Tens of thousands of South Korean soldiers were captured by the North Korean and Chinese forces during the war (1950–53) but were not returned during the prisoner exchanges under the 1953 Armistice Agreement. Most are presumed dead, but the South Korean government estimates that (as of 2007) some 560 South Korean prisoners of war still survive in North Korea.[7] The issue of unaccounted for South Korean POWs from the Korean War has been in dispute since the Armistice in 1953.

North Korea did not recognize the POW status of its South Korean captives, but viewed them as "liberated fighters." Because of this fundamental difference in perspective, captured South Korean soldiers were treated very differently from other UN captives.

Articles 49 through 57 of the 1949 Geneva Convention III specifically restrict the use of POW labor for military purposes. However, it was common practice to enlist former South Korean volunteers into North Korean forces after several weeks of re-education.

After the war, the former South Korean POWs were given North Korean citizenship after formally being discharged from their camps and units. Most of them were assigned to work in coal mines near their camps. Although they were nominally full citizens, they faced much discrimination in their employment and residence.

Beginning in 1951, the Chinese, alarmed by the excessive death rate, tried to improve the treatment of POWs. The Chinese recognized the propaganda value of POWs and established permanent POW camps in the far North, close to the Yalu River. The Chinese forces also held indoctrination sessions which many US prisoners charged was attempted brainwashing.

Red Cross inspections revealed that, in general, the North Korean POWs received wraps, bedding, and the standard ration for North Korean troops: rice or rice flour, barley, fish or canned meat, seaweed leaf, and cigarettes. American prisoners, however, suffered horrific treatment. Of 7000 US POWs, 2800 (40 %) died in captivity. Diet and medical conditions were notoriously bad.[6]

Every rule promulgated by the Geneva Convention was broken when thousands of Americans died at the hands of the Communists. American prisoners of war who were not deliberately murdered at the time of capture or shortly thereafter were starved, beaten, wounded, and tortured, or molested. They were displayed and humiliated before the civilian populace or forced to march long distances to Communist prison camps without adequate food, water, shelter, clothing, or medical care, and there to experience further acts of human indignities. The massacres and wholesale extermination of their victims was a calculated part of Communist psychological warfare.

Between 5000 and 7000 civilians as well as soldiers of the Republic of Korea, were also slaughtered at Taejon between September 23 and 27, 1950. On September 27, approximately 60 American prisoners who had been confined in Taejon prison were taken into the prison yard in groups of 14 with their hands wired together. Forced to sit hunched in hastily dug ditches, they were then shot by North Korean troops at point blank range with American M-1 rifles using armor-piercing ammunition. Of the two seriously wounded survivors, only one lived to recount the horrifying details.

In late December 1950, five American airmen in a truck convoy were ambushed by North Korean forces. When their bodies were discovered soon thereafter by a South Korean patrol, it was revealed that their flesh had been punctured in as many as 20 different areas with heated, sharpened bamboo sticks. The torture was so fiendish that one perforation was sufficient to cause death.[6]

Vietnam War. The Vietnam War was an undeclared war in Vietnam, Laos, and Cambodia beginning November 1, 1955, and ending with the fall of Saigon on April 30, 1975. North Vietnam was supported by the Soviet Union, China, and other communist allies; South Vietnam was allied to the United States, South Korea, the Philippines, Australia, Thailand, and other anticommunist nations. By 1964, there were 23,000 US troops in Vietnam. The conflict was further escalated by the 1964 Gulf of Tonkin incident. Up until then, it was the longest war in US history.

Members of the US armed forces were held as prisoners of war in significant numbers from 1964 to 1973. Unlike service members captured in World War II and the Korean War, who had been mostly enlisted troops, the overwhelming majority of Vietnam-era POWs were officers, most of them Navy, Air Force, and Marine Corps airmen. Most US prisoners were captured and held in North Vietnam by the North Vietnamese Army (NVA); a much smaller number were captured in the south and held by the National Liberation Front (Việt Cộng). A handful of American civilians was also held captive during the war.

The most widely known facility used to house US prisoners in North Vietnam was the Hỏa Lò Prison (nicknamed the "Hanoi Hilton"). The treatment and ultimate fate of US prisoners of war in Vietnam became a subject of widespread concern in the United States, and hundreds of thousands of Americans wore bracelets with the name and capture dates of imprisoned POWs.

American POWs in North Vietnam were released in early 1973 as part of Operation Homecoming, the result of diplomatic negotiations concluding US military involvement in Vietnam. After Operation Homecoming, the United States still listed roughly 1350 Americans as prisoners of war or missing in action and sought the return of roughly 1200 Americans reported killed in action but whose bodies had not been recovered. These missing personnel would become the subject of the Vietnam War POW/MIA issue.[8]

The US practice of handing over NVA and Viet Cong prisoners to the South Vietnamese military, where the abuse of such prisoners was commonly known, may have contributed to the abuse of American POWs held by the NVA and Viet Cong as a means of retaliation.

On March 26, 1964, CPT Floyd James Thompson became the first US service member imprisoned during the Vietnam War when his Bird Dog observation plane was brought down by small arms fire. He would ultimately spend just short of 9 years in captivity, making him the longest-held POW in American history. American pilots continued to be captured over the north between 1965 and 1968 during Operation Rolling Thunder, the sustained aerial bombing campaign against North Vietnam. After President Lyndon Johnson initiated a bombing pause in 1968, President Richard Nixon resumed bombing in 1969.

Even though North Vietnam was a signatory of the Third Geneva Convention of 1949, which demanded "decent and humane treatment" of prisoners of war, beginning in late 1965, use of torture against US prisoners became severe. During the first 6 years in which US prisoners were held in North Vietnam, many experienced long periods of solitary confinement. Robinson Risner and James Stockdale, two senior officers who were the de facto leaders of the POWs, were held in solitary confinement for 3 and 4 years, respectively.

US prisoners of war in North Vietnam were subjected to extreme torture and malnutrition during their captivity, including rope binding, irons, beatings, and prolonged solitary confinement. About 20% of the total POW population were nonpilots: infantrymen and Special Forces soldiers captured, for the most part, in the field. These prisoners withstood indescribable hardships—kept in bamboo cages with their feet often held in wooden stocks, existing on a starvation diet of rice and water. Sanitary conditions were nonexistent, disease was widespread, medical care was rare, and a large number died. Red Cross visits were never permitted. One justification for this policy was that the North Vietnamese considered the war to be an undeclared belligerency and that US servicemen were "criminals" and "air pirates."

The aim of the torture was usually not to acquire military information but to break the will of the prisoners, both individually and as a group. The goal of the North Vietnamese was to acquire written or recorded statements from the prisoners criticizing US conduct of the war and praising North Vietnamese treatment of prisoners, for use as propaganda.

During one such event in 1966, Jeremiah Denton, a captured Navy pilot, was forced to appear at a televised press conference, where he famously blinked the word "T-O-R-T-U-R-E" with his eyes in Morse code, confirming to US intelligence that American prisoners were being harshly treated. Two months later, in what became known as the Hanoi March, 52 American prisoners of war were paraded through the streets of Hanoi before thousands of North

Vietnamese civilians, who beat them along the two-mile route with their guards largely unable to restrain the attacks.

In the end, North Vietnamese torture was sufficiently brutal and prolonged that virtually every American POW so subjected made a statement of some kind. As one later wrote of finally being forced to make an anti-American statement: "I had learned what we all learned over there: Every man has his breaking point. I had reached mine." Realizing this, the Americans' aim became to absorb as much torture as they could before giving in. One later described the internal code the POWs developed, and instructed new arrivals thus: "Take physical torture until you are right at the edge of losing your ability to be rational. At that point, lie, do, or say whatever you must do to survive. But you first must take physical torture."[9]

The POWs made extensive use of a tap code to communicate. It was introduced in June 1965 by four POWs held in the Hỏa Lò: CPT Carlyle "Smitty" Harris had remembered the code from prior training and taught it to his fellow prisoners. In addition to allowing communication between walls, the prisoners used the code when sitting next to each other but forbidden from speaking by tapping on one another's bodies. Throughout the war, the tap code was instrumental in maintaining prisoner morale. During periods of protracted isolation, the tap code facilitated elaborate mental projects designed to preserve the prisoners' sanity.[7]

During the Johnson administration when a few captured servicemen began to be released from North Vietnamese prisons, their testimonies revealed the widespread and systematic abuse of the prisoners. Initially, this information was downplayed by American authorities for fear that conditions might worsen for those remaining in North

Vietnamese custody. The policy changed under the Nixon administration, when mistreatment of the prisoners was publicized by US Secretary of Defense Secretary Melvin Laird and others.

Beginning in October 1969, the torture regime suddenly abated to a great extent, and life for the prisoners became less severe and generally more tolerable, possibly due to the death of North Vietnamese leader Ho Chi Minh the previous month. Also, a badly beaten and weakened POW who had been released that summer disclosed to the world press the conditions to which the prisoners were being subjected, and the National League of Families of American Prisoners and Missing in Southeast Asia heightened awareness of the POWs' plight.

Despite several escape attempts, no US prisoner of war successfully escaped from a North Vietnamese prison. Although the November 1970 US Special Forces attempt to rescue 61 POWs believed to be held at the Sơn Tây prison camp failed, the mission had several positive implications for American prisoners. The most immediate effect was to affirm to the POWs that their government was actively attempting to repatriate them, which significantly boosted their morale.

By 1971, some 30%–50% of the POWs had become disillusioned about the war, both because of the apparent lack of military progress and in response to what they heard about the growing antiwar movement in the United States, and as a result, some of them were less reluctant to make propaganda statements for the North Vietnamese.

At the Hanoi Hilton, POWs cheered the resumed bombing of North Vietnam starting in April 1972, whose targets included the Hanoi area. The old-timers among the POWs cheered even more during the intense "Christmas

Bombing" campaign of December 1972, when Hanoi was subjected for the first time to repeated B-52 Stratofortress raids. Although its explosions lit the night sky and shook the walls of the camp, scaring some of the newer POWs, most saw it as a forceful measure to compel North Vietnam to finally come to terms.[7]

The most famous of Vietnam War prisoners of War was John S. McCain III, son of John S. McCain Jr, an admiral. His status as POW made the front pages of major American newspapers. While on a bombing mission during Operation Rolling Thunder over Hanoi in October 1967, he was shot down, seriously injured, and captured by the North Vietnamese. He was a prisoner of war until 1973, experiencing episodes of torture and refusing an out-of-sequence early release. During the war, he sustained wounds that left him with lifelong physical disabilities. He later became a US senator and presidential candidate.[10]

The Gulf War. The Gulf War was triggered by Iraq's invasion of Kuwait in August 1990 and brought into play the assistance of 35 nations, calling themselves The Coalition. For the first time, captivity issues were brought before the public on television.

The Coalition captured 86,743 Iraqis, compared with only 20 Americans, 12 Britons, 9 Saudis, 2 Italians, and 1 Kuwaiti (a pilot) taken prisoner by the Iraqis.[11] Of 23 US POWs, including two servicewomen, all were tortured or abused by their Iraqi captors. In some instances, interrogators broke bones, perforated eardrums, and threatened to shoot or dismember American prisoners. One of the women, a flight surgeon, was raped by one of her captors.[9]

Army colonel Bill Jordan said that Iraqi captors used "threats of death . . . beatings and/or electric shock" against American POWs. One Air Force captain was allegedly tortured by the Iraqi secret police by breaking his nose, dislocating his shoulder, and puncturing his eardrum. Two other captives were forced to make statements against the war in front of TV cameras, including the assertion that they had been wrong in attacking Iraqi civilians. They were also threatened to be used as human shields. Articles 3 and 13, respectively, of the Geneva Convention expressly forbid both these degradations.

Iraqi prisoners could not be used in bargaining for the return of Coalition prisoners because not only did Saddam Hussein not want them back—many of them did not want to return. Red Cross representatives were denied access to Coalition prisoners in Iraq.[12]

REFERENCES FOR CHAPTER VI

1   Vourkoutiotis V. World War II—Western Europe. In Vance JF, Ed. *Encyclopedia of Prisoners of War and Internment.* Santa Barbara, Calif: ABC-CLIO; 2000:341-342.

2   Burleigh M. The Third Reich: a New History. New York: Hill & Wang; 2000:518.

3   Zagovic RA. World War II—Eastern Front. In Vance JF, 329-333.

4   La Forte RS. World War II—Far East. In Vance JF, 333-336.

5   Prisoner-of-war camp: Conditions in Japanese camps. Available at: https://en.wikipedia.org/wiki/Prisoner-of-war_camp#Conditions_in_Japanese_camps. Accessed September 12, 2018.

6   German prisoners of war in the United States. Available at: https://en.wikipedia.org/wiki/German_prisoners_of_war_in_the_United_States. Accessed September 28, 2018.

7   Korean War POWs detained in North Korea. Available at: https://en.wikipedia.org/wiki/Korean_War_POWs_detained_in_North_Korea. Accessed October 3, 2018.

8   Reeder, WS Jr. Vietnam War (1959-1975). In Vance, 303-305.

9   Zink D. *Vietnam: Gone but Not Forgotten.* Bloomington, IN: Booktango; 2015: ch 5.

10 John McCain. Available at: https://en.wikipedia.org/wiki/John_McCain. Accessed May 18, 2019.

11 Vance JF. The Gulf War (1990-1991). In Vance, 123-124.

12 Healy M. (1991). Pentagon details abuse of American POWs in Iraq. *Los Angeles Times.* Available at: https://www.latimes.com/archives/la-xpm-1991-08-02-mn-223-story.html. Accessed October 24, 2019.

VII

POWS OF OTHER WARS

FRANCO-PRUSSIAN WAR (1870-71)

This was the last war of German unification, leading to the founding of the German Empire. The Imperial French Army was poorly led and was plagued with epidemics, especially in forts—the main line of defense. When the Sedan and Metz fortresses surrendered in September and October 1870, respectively, after only a few weeks of siege, they delivered huge numbers of POWs—totaling some 273,000 French—pretty much foretelling the outcome of the war.

Despite the great numbers of French prisoners, the Germans did their best to take care of them. France's most important prisoner, Emperor Napoleon III, was interned in Wilhelmshöhe Castle. Most of the captives enjoyed relative freedom. The officers captured at Sedan were released and sent home after giving their word of honor that they would not again bear arms against Germany. This was one of the practices originating in feudal times, which was mixed with more modern practices such as volunteer irregulars (*franc-tireurs*).

The rank and file complained that—besides homesickness and boredom—there was a lack of white bread and wine. Although there were epidemics, the death toll was acceptably low: less than 4%. Prisoners were rarely forced to labor since, first, the cold weather was coming on and, second, the idea did not appeal to industrialists.

The large number of prisoners taken by the Germans created a logistical challenge that turned out to be a harbinger of future wars. By war's end, French prisoners totaled 383,860 men. In addition, humanitarian arrangements between the powers, such as organized medical and Red Cross services, led to the enactment of POW treatment in the Hague conventions of 1899 and 1907.[1]

THE BOER WAR (1899-1902)

Fought between Great Britain and the two Boer (Afrikaner) republics, the South African Republic (Transvaal) and the Orange Free State, from 1899 to 1902. The South African War was caused by the refusal of the Boer leader Paul Kruger to grant political rights to the (mostly) English subjects in the interior mining districts and the aggressiveness of the British commissioner, Sir Alfred Milner.

It was during the early phases of the war that Winston Churchill first came to international attention when he escaped from a Boer prison. Although he was not in the military at the time (he was a war correspondent), Churchill was held in a POW camp. After only 4 weeks' captivity, he successfully escaped by scaling a wall that was out of the guards' sight. The Boers put a price on Churchill's head to be captured dead or alive. He returned to Britain as a celebrity and started on his path to becoming prime minister of the United Kingdom.

The Boers relied on guerrilla warfare, destroying railroads, cutting telegraph lines, and attacking isolated British outposts—always staying one step ahead of their lumbering pursuers. The British response was to set up complex nets of block houses, strong points, and barbed wire fences, partitioning off the entire conquered territory. In addition, civilian farms and live stock were destroyed in a scorched earth strategy. Survivors were forced into the Brits' own version of "concentration" camps. Over 26,000 women and children were to perish in these camps.

When Field Marshall Herbert Kitchener took over in late 1900, he introduced new tactics in an attempt to flush out the guerrillas in a series of systematic drives, organized like a sporting shoot, with success defined in terms of a weekly "bag" of killed, captured, and wounded, and to sweep the country bare of everything that could give sustenance to the guerrillas, including women and children. It was the clearance of civilians—uprooting a whole nation—that would come to dominate the last phase of the war.

The Boer War concentration camp system was the first time that a whole nation had been systematically targeted, and the first in which whole regions had been depopulated. Of the 28,000 Boer men captured as prisoners of war, 25,630 were sent overseas as there was nowhere that was suitable in South Africa. There, they were either freed or enslaved within civil societies. The vast majority of Boers remaining in the local camps were women and children.

The most notorious execution of prisoners was the killing of 12 Boer captives by the (Australian) Bushveldt Carbineers. Its officers (one of whom was the now-famous

Harry "Breaker" Morant) were court-marshaled and put to death by firing squad.

The camps were poorly administered from the outset and became increasingly overcrowded when Kitchener's troops implemented the internment strategy on a vast scale. Furthermore, the neglect, poor hygiene, and bad sanitation led to malnutrition and endemic contagious diseases such as measles, typhoid, and dysentery to which the children were particularly vulnerable. Coupled with a shortage of modern medical facilities, many of the internees died.

These conditions might have gone on indefinitely had it not been for Emily Hobhouse, a British welfare campaigner, who brought them to the attention of the British public and worked to change the deprived conditions inside the concentration camps, as well as to raise public awareness in Europe of the atrocities. By then it was too late, however, for the 28,000 Boers and the more than 14,000 Africans who died in the camps, most of them women and children.[2]

RUSSO-JAPANESE WAR (1904-1905)

This was the first major conflict in recent years in the time period between European and Asian combatants. It changed the balance of power in Asia, setting the stage for World War I, and was especially noteworthy for the generous treatment of POWs. President Theodore Roosevelt won the Nobel Peace Prize for mediating the Portsmouth Peace Treaty at war's end.

Approximately 70,000 Russian sailors and soldiers were captured and only 1728 Japanese. Although the latter would have to apologize and endure insults, they were seldom punished harshly. Only a few officers were forced to resign.

However, treatment by both sides was commendable in every respect. In an effort to demonstrate its humanitarian spirit, the Japanese instituted regulations conforming with the recently signed Hague Convention of 1899, which called for parole walks for officers, roomy barracks, free postage, and the exchange or release of sick or wounded prisoners. POWs who were transported to a camp in Masuyama were encouraged to read and write Japanese and to walk freely around the city, although there were exceptions to this benevolence: When the Japanese discovered thousands of drunken Russian soldiers at Mukden, in a forewarning of things to come, instead of capturing them, they clubbed and disemboweled them with bayonets.

However, this compassionate treatment may have had unintended consequences: First, these incidents set the stage for later prohibitions against surrender in later wars, and second, when the time came to revise the Hague Convention in 1907, some of the lawmakers felt that—based on the events of the Russo-Japanese War, sufficient protections were already in place. But World War I soon demonstrated how tragically short-sighted they were.[3]

THE RUSSIAN CIVIL WAR (1917–1922)

The Russian Civil War was a multiparty conflict in the former Russian Empire that occurred immediately after the two Russian Revolutions of 1917. It was one of the most bitter and costly internal conflicts in modern history.

The two largest combatant groups were the Red Army, led by Vladimir Lenin, fighting for the Bolshevik form of socialism, and the loosely allied forces known as the White Army, which included diverse interests favoring political monarchism, economic capitalism, and alternative forms of socialism. The Red Army eventually defeated the White Armed Forces of South Russia in Ukraine and the army led by Admiral Aleksandr Kolchak to the east in Siberia in 1919. The remains of the White forces commanded by Pyotr Nikolayevich Wrangel were beaten in Crimea and evacuated in late 1920. An estimated 7 to12 million casualties occurred during the war, mostly civilians. The Russian Civil War has been described by some as the greatest national catastrophe that Europe had yet seen.[4]

Prisoners of war, as well as combatants, suffered from relentless hunger, disease, shortages, and deficient medical care. From the beginning, as central authority collapsed, the war was marked with extreme brutality. The treatment of prisoners by both sides was notoriously cruel and fickle. Many were shot or hanged without a trial. The Reds put POWs into forced labor camps where thousands died from disease, starvation, and mass shootings. Barbaric methods of execution—from drowning and crucifixion and live burials to immersion in boiling water—were used. Entire villages were burned down in retaliation for resistance or sympathy with the enemy. The violent excesses were a product of the deep ideological fervor fueling each side.[4]

SECOND SINO-JAPANESE WAR (1937-45)

Many historians consider this war to be a forerunner to World War II.

REFERENCES FOR CHAPTER VII

1   Nachtigal, R. Franco-Prussian War (1870-1871). In Vance JF, Ed. *Encyclopedia of Prisoners of War and Internment.* Santa Barbara, Calif: ABC-CLIO; 2000:102-103.
2   Second Boer War. Available at: https://en.wikipedia.org/wiki/Second_Boer_War#Concentration_cam....../.ps. Accessed May 8, 2019.
3   Vance JF. Russo-Japanese War. In Vance JF; 2000:259-260.
4   McLarnand E. Russian Civil War. In Vance JF; 2000:258-259.

VIII

THE SELECTEES

HOW WERE THEY SELECTED? (THE 12)

As the title of this book suggests, these men were selected on the basis of going beyond the call of duty. As dental officers, their duty was to address the dental—and often the medical—needs of their fellow soldiers (and sailors) of their command.

But the exigencies of war demand that patient care sometimes be subordinated to more pressing needs. The dental surgeon must remember that he or she is first, a soldier or sailor and second, a dentist.

In some cases, my interpretation of "above the call of duty" was somewhat liberal. For example, Albert Brown's entitlement as a selectee was that he was the longest-lived survivor of the Death March, living to 105. Strictly speaking, surviving the Death March was only in the line of duty. However, I think such a feat (and there were others on his part) deserves recognition.

Varaztad Kazanzian was only doing his job when he performed his "miracle" surgery, but think of the number of faces he made whole! Surely Coenraad Moorrees, who administered to his fellow prisoners of war (POWs) while he himself suffered from multiple maladies warrants mention. And the fact that he became a consummate orthodontic educator only adds to his stature.

What makes an ordinarily peace-loving dentist, when confronted with the circumstances of war, rise to the occasion and perform acts of heroism, as exemplified by these twelve dental officers, all of whom, in order to qualify for selection, needed three qualifications, as mentioned in the Preface: (1) They each had a DDS or DMD, (2) they were members of the armed forces, and (3) their feats were performed during time of war (WWI or WWII).

In keeping with the historical nature of this account, the selectees are grouped by wars. Three carried out their exploits during World War I, one served in both world wars, and the other eight were involved in World War II. Of these eight, six were POWs; two were not. Of the six POWs, three were American, two were Scottish, and one was Dutch-American.

WORLD WAR I—UNITED STATES

HE RECEIVED THE MEDAL OF HONOR

(one of two Navy dental officers to do so) for saving the life of a Marine corporal under fire.

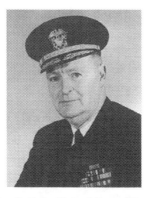

Alexander G. Lyle. United States Navy Photo.

Alexander Gordon Lyle was born in Gloucester, Mass, on November 12, 1889. After graduating from high school, he went to Baltimore College, graduating in 1912 with a degree in dentistry. He accepted a commission in the Navy as a LTJG in 1915.

Lyle was serving as a dental officer with the 5th Regiment of the US Marine Corps on the French front during World War I. On April 23, 1918, he risked his life to rescue a corporal who had been seriously wounded during heavy shell fire. He saved the corporal's life by treating his wounds and became one of only three dental officers in history to receive the Medal of Honor. At the time the award was made, the Navy still had two different versions of the medal, one for combat operations and one for noncombat operations. For his actions in saving the corporal's life, Lyle received the combat version of the medal, known as the Tiffany Cross.

His citation reads:

> For extraordinary heroism and devotion to duty while serving with the 5th Regiment, U.S. Marine Corps. Under heavy shellfire, on April

> 23, 1918, on the French Front, Lt. Comdr. Lyle
> rushed to the assistance of Cpl. Thomas Regan,
> who was seriously wounded, and administered
> such effective surgical aid while bombardment
> was still continuing, as to save the life of Cpl.
> Regan.

Lyle's medal can be seen on display at the National Naval Medical Center, Bethesda, Maryland. In addition to the MOH, Lyle also received the Legion of Merit, the Silver Star (with palms), and the Italian War Cross. Between wars, he was attached to the 4th Marines in China. From 1932 to '36, he was chief of dental service at Newport Naval Hospital in Rhode Island. Two years into WWII, he was promoted to rear admiral and appointed chief of the Navy Dental Corps, the first Navy dentist to achieve flag rank. In 1946, he was awarded the doctor of science degree. In 1947 after 32 years of service, he was promoted to vice admiral (VADM) on the retired list. He died in 1955 and was buried in Arlington National Cemetery.[4]

Medal of Honor

The Congressional Medal of Honor is the highest military commendation our government can bestow, reserved for those who have "distinguished themselves conspicuously by gallantry and intrepidity." It is usually conferred by the President.

The first Medals of Honor were presented to six members of the group known as "Andrews' Raiders" by Civil-War-era Secretary of War Edwin M. Stanton on March 25,

1863, during the Civil War, in recognition of their voluntary participation in the "Great Locomotive Chase" deep within Confederate lines. As of October 17, 2018, 3522 Medals of Honor have been awarded American servicemen.[3]

HE WAS THE SECOND DENTAL OFFICER TO RECEIVE THE MEDAL OF HONOR

(posthumously) for rescuing under fire his wounded commanding officer.

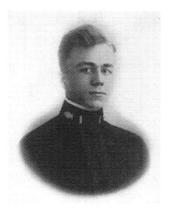

Weedon Edward Osborne. Public Domain. Credit: Naval History & Heritage Command

Six years after the founding of the Navy Dental Corps, the United States entered World War I. Dental Corps personnel were deployed on ships and attached to Marine Corps units, where they served on the front lines with distinction. One such dental officer was LTJG Weedon E. Osborne, who was born in Chicago (November 13, 1892) and graduated from Northwestern University Dental School in 1915. On March 30, 1918, he was appointed as a Navy dental surgeon, reporting to the Sixth Marine Regiment. Two months later, he was on the front lines as an assistant surgeon for the 96th Company, commanded by CPT Donald F. Duncan. During the battle of Belleau Wood on June 6, 1918, Duncan received orders to attack the village of Bouresches, France. The company advanced following an artillery barrage that proved ineffectual, and the Marines were thrashed with mortar and heavy machine gun fire. Osborne paid little heed, repeatedly rescuing Marines and tending to their wounds. Although his profession gave him every justification for remaining in the rear, he volunteered for general rescue work and aided the wounded.[1]

Duncan was leading a charge when he was struck in the abdomen by machine gun fire. Osborne and two others carried their severely wounded captain to a nearby grove of trees. They had no sooner set Duncan down when an artillery shell exploded nearby, killing Duncan, Osborne, and one other Marine. For his heroism, Osborne was awarded the Medal of Honor (MOH) posthumously. He also received the Army's Distinguished Cross and the Purple Heart. The MOH citation reads:

> For extraordinary heroism while attached to the 6th Regiment, US Marines, in actual conflict with the enemy and under fire during the advance on Bouresches, France, on 6 June 1918. In the hottest of the fighting when the Marines made their famous advance on Bouresches at the southern edge of Belleau Wood, LTJG Osborne threw himself zealously into the work of rescuing the wounded. Extremely courageous in the performance of this perilous task, he was

killed while carrying a wounded officer to a
place of safety.

He was the first commissioned officer of the US Navy
to be killed in action during land fighting overseas.[1] The
destroyer USS *Osborne* and the headquarters of the 2nd
Dental Company at Camp Lejeune were named for him,
as was the USS *Osborne* Dental Clinic in North Chicago,
Illinois.[2]

"THE MIRACLE MAN OF THE WESTERN FRONT"

was the moniker given Varaztad H. Kazanjian, an Armenian
American dentist commissioned in the British Dental
Corps, for the reconstructive facial surgery he performed
on "hopelessly" disfigured soldiers during World War One.

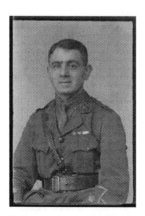

Dr. Varaztad H. Kazanjian in WWI uniform as British
dental officer. Courtesy of Kazanjian family.

Varaztad H. Kazanjian was born in Erzincan, Ottoman
Empire, on March 18, 1879, where he attended a French

Jesuit school in the city of Sivas. Thereafter, he moved to Samsun to live with his older half-brother. While in Samsun, he first worked with his brother but eventually moved to a position in a post office. In an attempt to escape the massacres of Armenians in his country, he left for the United States in October 1895 and settled in Worcester, Mass, taking a job in the local wire factory. It was at the mill that Kazanjian first displayed the natural dexterity that would serve him well in the field of plastic surgery.

Because he understood neither English nor the procedure, his first week's pay in America was 90 cents. Two weeks later, as he quickly learned the routine, it had risen to $6. His desire for knowledge was so strong that he began night school immediately upon his arrival in Worcester— not missing a class for 7 years. He became an avid reader, took correspondence courses, and was privately tutored in English, often at the end of a 10-hour workday. He was finally awarded the DMD degree in 1905 by Harvard University.

Kazanjian opened his first dental office in Boston— modest in both proportions and patronage. With time on his hands, he began a lifetime teaching career at Harvard. In the clinic, he treated more than 400 cases of jaw fracture, being one of the first to eliminate the clumsy splint and substitute the simpler intermaxillary wiring. His years at the wire mill had paid off. He also fabricated artificial noses, eyes, and ears for patients who had lost tissues to injury or cancer surgery. As his reputation grew, dentists began referring difficult cases to him. In 1912, he was appointed head of Harvard's Prosthetic Laboratory.

Soon after WWI broke out, a group of American universities, Harvard at the lead, undertook to staff a much-needed base hospital at Carniers, France, to care for casualties of the British Expeditionary Forces. Known as the First Harvard Unit, it consisted of 32 physicians and surgeons, 75 nurses, and 3 dentists, one of whom was Dr. Kazanjian. In 1915, he was appointed chief dental officer of the unit. Here he established the first dental and maxillofacial unit in France, where he treated some of the most serious injuries suffered in trench warfare—jaws, noses, cheeks, and skulls shattered by bullets and grenades. Few clinicians were prepared to treat the avalanche of broken faces that only increased as the war dragged on. Recognizing that deficiency—even in England where specialized treatment facilities were nonexistent—Kazanjian took it upon himself to treat these unfortunates.

Working under primitive conditions in makeshift hospitals near the battlefields, Kazanjian exhibited the humane concern combined with innovative medical procedures that established his reputation and marked his subsequent career as a founder of the modern practice of plastic surgery. He was eventually dubbed the "Miracle Man of the Western Front." In June 1916, he was promoted to the rank of major and made a Companion of the Order of St Michael and St George by King George of England.

Returning to Boston after the war, Dr Kazanjian realized that, without the MD degree, he could not legally carry out the same surgical procedures he had performed in France. So, at age 40, he matriculated at Harvard's medical school. Soon after graduating, he was named professor of clinical oral surgery at Harvard University. He continued in his private practice well into his '80s. His honors and awards are too numerous to mention, but they include an honorary degree from Emerson College (his favorite?) received in a combined ceremony with his niece, Arlene Francis, who was a movie actress, radio and TV personality, and long-time hostess of the TV series, *What's My Line?*

Varaztad Kazanjian will be remembered not only for his medical innovations, but for his modesty and kindness.[5]

OTHER ALLIED COUNTRIES

HE FOUGHT IN TWO WORLD WARS

under two flags, was wounded nine times, and was decorated for performing a swimming feat under Turkish fire at Gallipoli.

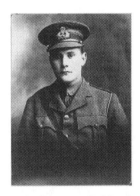

Bernard G. Freyberg. Public domain.

Bernard Cyril Freyberg was born in Richmond, Surrey, UK, to James Freyberg and his second wife, Julia (née Hamilton). He moved to New Zealand (NZ) with his parents at the age of two and attended Wellington College from 1897 to 1904. A strong swimmer, he won the NZ 100-yard championship in 1906 and 1910.

In May 1911, Freyberg gained formal registration as a dentist. He worked as an assistant dentist in Morrinsville and later practiced in Hamilton and in Levin. Freyberg left NZ in March 1914. According to a 1942 *Life* magazine article, Freyberg went to San Francisco and Mexico around this time, and was a captain under Pancho Villa during the Mexican Revolution. Upon learning of the outbreak of war in Europe in August 1914, he traveled to Britain via Los Angeles (where he won a swimming competition) and New York (where he won a prizefight), to earn money to cross the United States and the Atlantic.

Volunteering for service in England, Fryberg joined the 7th "Hood" Battalion of the Royal Naval Brigade, and he was on the Belgian front in September 1914. In late 1914 Freyberg met Winston Churchill, then First Lord of the Admiralty. He persuaded Churchill to grant him a Royal Naval Volunteer Reserve commission in the battalion, part of the 2nd (Royal Naval) Brigade of the newly constituted Royal Naval Division.

In April 1915 Freyberg became involved in the Dardanelles campaign. On the night of 24 April, during the initial landings by Allied troops following the failed naval attempt to force the straits by sea, Freyberg volunteered to swim ashore via the Gulf of Saros. Once there, he began lighting flares so as to distract the defending Turkish forces from the real landings taking place at Gallipoli. Despite coming under heavy Turkish fire, he returned safely from this outing and was awarded the Distinguished Service Order (DSO) for his achievements. He received serious wounds on several occasions and left the peninsula when his division evacuated in January 1916.

In May 1916, Freyberg was transferred to the British Army as a captain in the Queen's (Royal West Surrey) Regiment. He remained with the Hood Battalion, however, as a seconded temporary major and went with them to France.

During the final stages of the Battle of the Somme, while commanding a battalion as a temporary lieutenant colonel, he so distinguished himself in the capture of Beaucourt village that he was awarded the Victoria Cross.

On November 13, 1916, at Beaucourt-sur-Ancre, France, after Freyberg's battalion had carried the initial attack through the enemy's front system of trenches, he rallied and re-formed his own much disorganized unit and, adding some additional men, led the unit on a successful assault on the second objective. During the battle, he suffered two wounds, but remained in command and held his ground throughout the day and the following night. When reinforced the next morning, he attacked and captured a strongly fortified village, taking 500 prisoners. Although wounded twice more, the second time severely, Freyberg refused to leave the line until he had issued final instructions. The citation for his DSO award, published in the *London Gazette*, reads

> The personality, valour and utter contempt of danger on the part of this single Officer enabled the lodgment in the most advanced objective of the Corps to be permanently held, and on this point d'appui the line was eventually formed. During his time on the Western Front Freyberg continued to lead by example. His bold leadership had a cost: Freyberg received nine wounds during his service in France, and men who served with him later in his career said hardly a part of his body did not have scars.[6]

Freyberg gained promotion to the rank of temporary brigadier general (BG; although he still had only the permanent rank of captain) and took command of the

173rd Brigade in April 1917, which reportedly made him the youngest general officer in the British Army. He was awarded a Companion of the Order of St Michael and St George the same year. In September, a shell exploding at his feet inflicted the worst of his many wounds.

Freyberg ended his war experience by leading a cavalry squadron detached from 7th Dragoon Guards to seize a bridge at Lessines, which was achieved one minute before the armistice came into effect, thus earning him a second bar to the DSO. By the end of the war, Freyberg had added the French Croix de Guerre to his name, as well receiving five mentions in dispatches after his escapade at Saros. With his VC and three DSOs, he ranked among the most highly decorated British Empire soldiers of the First World War.

Early in 1919, Freyberg was granted a Regular Army commission in the Grenadier Guards and settled into peacetime soldiering, as well as continued attempts to swim the English Channel. He attended the Staff College, Camberley, from 1920 to 1921. From 1921 to 1925 he was a staff officer at the headquarters of the 44th (Home Counties) Division. He suffered health problems arising from his many wounds, and as part of his convalescence he visited NZ in 1921. On June 14, 1922, he married Barbara McLaren who had two children from her previous marriage; she and Freyberg later had a son, Paul (1923–1993).

During the '20s and '30s, Freyburg rose steadily in rank until July 1934, when he was promoted to major general (MG). During these years, he wrote *A Study of Unit Administration*, which became a staff college textbook on quartermasters' logistics; it went into a second edition in 1940. With his promotion at age 45, he seemed headed for the highest echelons of the army. Unfortunately, however, medical examinations prior to a posting to India revealed a heart problem. Despite strenuous efforts to surmount this, Freyberg was obliged to retire on 16 October 1937, after being classified as unfit for active service.

However, after the outbreak of war in September 1939, he was reinstated to the active list the following December as a specially employed major general. On being approached by the NZ government, Freyberg offered his services and was appointed commander of the 2nd New Zealand Expeditionary Force and of the 2nd NZ Division, leading their campaigns in Greece, North Africa, and Italy. In the chaos of the retreat from the Battle of Greece in 1941, Churchill gave Freyberg command of the Allied forces during the Battle of Crete. Although instructed to prevent an assault from the air, he remained obsessed with the (highly improbable) possibility of a naval landing and based his tactics on it, neglecting to adequately defend the airfield at Maleme, and ignoring ULTRA intelligence messages, which showed that the assault was coming by air.

Despite Freyberg's failure to prepare for an airborne assault and his defeat within 12 days by the barest margin, his destruction of the German 7th Flieger Division resulted in Hitler's never considering an operational airborne assault again. Although accepting responsibility for the defeat, Freyberg should not be held entirely culpable for the loss of Crete. Poor tactical leadership by Freyberg's subordinate commanders and their failure to prosecute his operational plan, in addition to their lack of sufficient weapons, communications, and transport contributed to the defeat.[7]

Although Freyberg was criticized for the destruction of the Benedictine Monastery above Cassino in 1944, he was admired for his concern for his men's welfare and for his willingness to serve at the forefront of enemy action. During this war, a third bar was added to his DSO and he was promoted to lieutenant general. He was also appointed as Knight Commander to the Most Excellent Order of the British Empire and the Most Honourable of the Bath, the latter for his leadership during the decisive battle at El Alamein, which marked a turning point for the Allies.

After the war, Freyberg was asked to serve as governor-general of NZ, the first such officer with a NZ upbringing. During this service, he was instrumental in compiling an official war history. His term was extended from 5 to 6 years due to an impending royal visit, among other reasons.

Following his return to England in August 1952, he frequently sat in the House of Lords, having been elevated to the peerage the previous year. From 1953 until his death, he served as deputy constable and lieutenant governor in charge of Windsor Castle, where he died on July 4, 1963, after the rupture of one of his war wounds. Dentist, athlete, soldier in two world wars, Bernard Freyberg could always be found in the thick of things.[8]

REFERENCES FOR CHAPTER VIII

1   Hyson JM Jr, Whitehorne JWA, Geenwood JT. *A History of Dentistry in the US Army to World War II*. Washington, DC: Office of the Surgeon General. Borden Institute; 2008: 621.

2   Weedon Osborne. Available at: https://en.wikipedia.org/wiki/Weedon_Osborne. Accessed April 1, 2018.

3   Marsh A. POWs in American History: a Synopsis. https://www.nps.gov/ande/learn/historyculture/pow_synopsis.htm. Updated 1998. Accessed January 10, 2020.

4   Alexander Gordon Lyle. Available at: https://en.wikipedia.org/wiki/Alexander_Gordon_Lyle. Accessed November 12, 2018.

5   Varaztad Kazanjian. Available at: https://en.wikipedia.org/wiki/Varaztad_Kazanjian. Accessed June 8, 2019.

6   Untitled. *The London Gazette (Supplement)*. December 15, 1916. p. 12307.

7   Bliss J. *The Fall of Crete 1941: Was Freyberg Culpable?* [Master's thesis]. Fort Leavenworth, Kansas: US Army Command and General Staff College, 2006; 159 pp.

8   Bernard Freyberg, 1st Baron Freyberg. Retrieved from: https://en.wikipedia.org/wiki/Bernard_Freyberg,_1st_Baron_Freyberg. Accessed June 30, 2019.

IX

THE SELECTEES— WWII—US—POWS

HE PERFORMED FERRYING AND GUERRILLA ACTIVITIES

behind enemy lines in the Mediterranean and was tortured as a POW, but his postwar testimony helped expose Nazi atrocities.

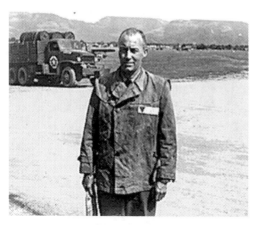

LCDR Jack Hedrick Taylor. Courtesy William McVay.

Jack Hedrick Taylor was born in Manhattan, Kansas, in 1908, son of John E. Taylor, an orthodontist. When Jack was a child, the family moved to Hollywood, California, where Dr Taylor set up a practice. Seeking to follow in his father's footsteps, Jack received a dental degree from USC in1932 and an orthodontics certificate in 1936.

He chose Santa Monica as a practice location so he could be close to his true love, the sea. He owned a number of boats and served as navigator on several yacht races to Hawaii and Bermuda. When the United States entered WWII, he refused a commission as a dental officer in favor of combat duty in the Navy.[1,2]

When it was learned that Taylor could handle small boats and even had done some exploring of the Channel Islands, he was transferred to the Office of Strategic Services (OSS) to participate in possible landings on enemy shores. He became chief instructor of the Area D Maritime School, specializing in navigation, seamanship, sailing, rowing, and night exercises. Promoted to chief of the OSS Maritime Unit, he personally commanded 14 missions on the enemy-occupied Greek and Balkan coasts, delivering spies, weapons, explosives, and other supplies to Allied forces from fall 1943 to spring 1944.[1] On one of the missions, he was dive-bombed and strafed. In the fall of that year, Taylor volunteered for a dangerous parachute drop behind enemy lines with three Austrian NCOs (who had been liberated from a POW camp) to obtain vital data on targets for the Air Corps. It was on this jump that Taylor satisfied the "air" requirement of a sea, air, and land (S-E-A-L) commando to become the first US service member to engage in commando missions in all three arenas.[1] He is thus considered the first Navy SEAL, although his military service preceded the actual formation of the unit by nearly 20 years.

He was captured by the Gestapo, taken to a Vienna prison, where his arm was broken, and he was placed in solitary confinement. In March 1945, Taylor was transferred to Mauthausen–a death camp–and the execution annex of Dachau. No one is known to have survived it more than 2 months. Only two Americans did so: Taylor and one other. After about 6 weeks of starvation, beatings, and slave labor, he was scheduled for execution. Only through the friendly intervention of a Czech inmate, who removed Taylor's papers and burned them, did Taylor escape death. Two days before V-E Day, Taylor and 15,000 other inmates were liberated by LTG Patton's Third Army. His weight had dropped from 170 to 110 and despite his infirmities, Taylor insisted on remaining at Mathausen to gather what was, according to Navy estimates, "probably the best single collection of firsthand evidence on war crimes . . ."

After the war, he was requested by President Truman to return to Europe to testify at the war crimes trials. His testimony helped convict some 58 Nazis to death. He was awarded the Navy Cross, a Bronze Star, the Distinguished Service Cross, and the Purple Heart.

Back home, Taylor took on a new interest: flying. He explored Mexico from the air and made plans to build a sportsman's lodge at the tip of Baja California. But his dream came to an end when his plane crashed on a routine flight. He died as he had lived: testing the elements, dueling with danger.[2]

Norman Wahl, DDS, MS, MA

THE MAUTHAUSEN CONCENTRATION
CAMP (1938–45)

On 12 March, 1938, the *Anschluss* (Annexation) of Austria to the German Reich took place. Two weeks later, the National Socialist *Gauleiter* (regional head) of Upper Austria, August Eigruber, announced to an enthusiastic audience that his district would have the "distinction" of building a concentration camp. The location chosen was the town of Mauthausen on the Danube River. Political opponents and groups of people labeled as "criminal'" or "antisocial" would be imprisoned here and forced to work in the granite quarries.

In August 1938 the SS transferred the first prisoners from the Dachau concentration camp. During this phase, the prisoners, who were all Germans and Austrians and all men, had to build their own camp and set up operations in the quarry. Their daily lives were shaped by hunger, arbitrary treatment, and violence. In December 1939 the SS ordered the construction of a second concentration camp just a few kilometers from Mauthausen—the Gusen branch camp.

After the outbreak of war, people from across Europe were deported to Mauthausen. During this phase, Mauthausen and Gusen were the concentration camps with the harshest imprisonment conditions and the highest mortality. Prisoners at the bottom of the camp hierarchy had little chance of surviving for long. Inmates were subjected to the most barbaric conditions imaginable, the most infamous of which was being forced to carry heavy stone blocks up 186 steps from the camp quarry. The steps became known as the "stairway to death." Those who were ill or otherwise useless to the SS were in constant danger of their lives. In 1941 the SS began construction of a gas chamber and other installations at Mauthausen for the systematic murder of large groups of people.

During the second half of the war, the prisoners, which now for the first time included women, were increasingly used as forced laborers in the arms industry. More and more, Mauthausen became a camp where the sick and weak were sent to die. Since the prisoners were now needed for their labor, living conditions improved for a short time. From the end of 1943 onward, inmates were also deployed in the construction of underground factories. The murderous working conditions that prevailed at these sites soon led to a dramatic rise in the number of deaths. Toward the end of the war, the Mauthausen concentration camp became the destination for evacuations from camps near the front line. Tens of thousands of prisoners arrived on several large transports. Overcrowding, lack of food, and rampant disease led to mass deaths among the prisoners in the final months before liberation.

On May 5, 1945, the 11th Armored Division of GEN Patton's Third US Army reached Gusen and Mauthausen and liberated the prisoners. Some prisoners were in such a weakened state that they died in the days and weeks after liberation. One of the survivors, Simon Wiesenthal, spent the rest of his life hunting down Nazi war criminals. Of a total of around 190,000 people imprisoned in the Mauthausen concentration camp and its subcamps over 7 years, at least 90,000 died.[3]

POW TREATMENT BY GERMANS VS JAPANESE

During World War II, which country was the most brutal toward POWs? The answer to that depends a great deal on who the POWs were. Generally speaking, the Western Powers both dispensed and received the most humane treatment. Another generalization involves the traditional German hatred of the Slavs (notably Russians), whom they considered subhuman.

A glance at the longevity data (used herein as a yardstick of brutality) will bear this out. Of the Russian prisoners held by the Germans, 57.5% died while in captivity. At the other extreme is the death rate of German POWs held by the British: 0.03%. To compare the treatment of British POWs by the Germans vs the Japanese, we can use the figures 3.5% vs 24.8%, respectively. There is no question that the Japanese were the most brutal. Thirty-three percent of American prisoners held by the Japanese died in captivity. Some estimates go as high as 40%. Only 0.001% of Chinese prisoners in China survived the war.

The Japanese were not always cruel. What made them change? In many respects, the Western Powers brought this savagery on themselves. During the first 30 years of the 20th century, the Japanese had shown wartime combatants exceptionally humane treatment. Their conduct during the Boxer Rebellion (1900), when they were part of the international military force that rescued Christians and Westerners from Peking, was exemplary. Even so, many Westerners called them "laughable yellow monkeys."

Trying to demonstrate that they were not an inferior people, they proved to be chivalrous in the 1904-05 war with Russia, rescuing the crews of torpedoed cruisers. Likewise, after the sea battle of Tsushima, rescued Russians were fed, clothed, and treated well. However, the Treaty of Portsmouth required the Japanese to withdraw from almost all the territories they won. The army was disgusted.

Japan abided by the Fourth Hague Convention (1907) after their entrance into World War I, and the Red Cross gave them high marks for their treatment of prisoners. As a member of the "Big Five" at the Paris peace conferences of 1919, however, Japan felt rejected when the Western powers refused to agree to ban racial discrimination, and, in 1921–22, at the Washington Naval Conference, Japan was relegated to a second-class naval power. After all these insults, it is no wonder that they began to see themselves as set apart and to declare themselves to be morally superior people.

Japan did sign the Geneva Convention but, like the USSR, failed to ratify it, so they were not bound by its laws. The 1929 Geneva Convention specified that POWs be treated humanely in all circumstances and to be protected against any act of violence, as well as against intimidation, insults, and public curiosity. However, .fighting the Chinese in 1930, the Japanese resorted to brutalities that they would never have engaged in a few years before. In World War II, they savagely brutalized thousands of American and Filipino POWs on the infamous Bataan Death March. Such cruelty may be explained by their belief that surrender was the ultimate shame; thus, POWs did not deserve humane treatment.[4]

AMERICAN POWS IN THE PACIFIC

Although dentists have been taken prisoner since the Civil War, it was not until World War II, when more than 22,000 dentists were serving in the armed forces, that any substantial number of them became at risk of becoming prisoners of war (POWs). In the case of the Pacific theatre, the total number of American military dentists captured during WWII was 53 (39 Army and 14 Navy).

With the defeat of troops in Bataan, Japan found itself in possession of 80,000 Philippine-American POWs. In order to relocate them from Bataan to complete the conquest of Corregidor, these prisoners endured one of the most infamous ordeals of human history—the Bataan Death March. Between 17,000 and 20,000 men (2300–4000 Americans) died on the march. Eight of the survivors were dentists. Remarkably, these eight not only survived the march but also the Camp O'Donnell "Death Camp" and the ensuing 40 months of imprisonment.

Two of these received bayonet wounds: Albert N. Brown (more about him later), while helping a fellow prisoner, and Denton J. Rees, for trying to salvage his medical supplies. Another dentist, Curtis E. Burson, attempted to save his dental instruments, but, according to his wife, "in the searing heat, with no water and no food, he gradually had to let them fall by the wayside."

Nor was there any relief when it was necessary to transport prisoners from one of the 650 camps scattered throughout the Pacific to another. On the contrary, their misery was only magnified. They were jammed into the hulls of cargo ships, aptly named "hell ships," spending weeks at sea with little food or water and horribly inadequate latrine facilities. These conditions only worsened as the war dragged on. Their captors failed to mark the vessels as carrying POWS, so as the Allies gained control of the seas, the hell ships came under increasing attack. When ships loaded with over 15,000 POWs were sunk by Allied planes or submarines, one could count on at least 10,000 fatalities.[5]

Hell Ships

In May 1942, the Japanese began transferring POWs by sea. Similar to treatment on the Bataan Death March, prisoners were often crammed into cargo holds with little air, food, or water for journeys that would last weeks. Many died from asphyxia, starvation, or dysentery. Some POWs became delirious and unresponsive in their environment of heat, humidity, and lack of oxygen, food, and water. These unmarked prisoner transports were targeted as enemy ships by Allied submarines and aircraft.

More than 20,000 Allied POWs died at sea when the transport ships carrying them were attacked by Allied submarines and aircraft. Although Allied headquarters often knew of the presence of POWs through radio interception and code breaking, the ships were sunk because interdiction of critical strategic materials was more important than the lives of prisoners-of-war and because Allied leaders feared that a pattern of sparing POW ships might lead the Japanese to use prisoners as human shields on valuable targets.

Norman Wahl, DDS, MS, MA

If the prisoners were lucky enough to survive the beatings, bayoneting, and infections, there was no escaping the effects of malnutrition. Weight loss was universal. The diet consisted almost entirely of rice (polished and of poor quality), so vitamin deficiency soon became widespread. Night blindness developed from lack of Vitamin A. Classical syndromes such as beriberi (due to thiamine deficiency) and a variety of more obscure neurological and dermatological syndromes appeared. Painful lower leg neuropathy (commonly known as "happy feet") was especially common.

"Wet" beriberi was characterized by cardiovascular failure and peripheral edema. The "dry" type resulted in foot or wrist drop. In its later stages, dry beriberi brought about sudden, sharp pains in the legs or feet, especially at night. One victim found that chewing tobacco brought relief.

Pellagra affected 50% of the POWs in moderate-to-severe form. A niacin (nicotinic acid) deficiency was seen in all four of its manifestations: dermatitis, diarrhea, dementia, and death. Of the nutritional skin syndromes, possibly the most unusual and distressing was scrotal dermatitis (probably due to riboflavin deficiency). It was manifested by inflammation, exudation, and swelling of the scrotal skin and was extremely uncomfortable.

Oral symptoms of pellagra were common. A physician POW observed that the "mucous membrane of the entire mouth and nasopharynx became inflamed. The tongue was a swollen, raw, beefy mass . . . crenelated by pressure against the teeth. Chewing and swallowing caused such extreme agony that the patient could only ingest small amounts of food or water."

Prisoners working almost naked in the jungle were particularly susceptible to tropical ulcers. Most were caused by bamboo scratches. A coworker reported, "Leg ulcers

118

of over a foot in length and maybe six inches in breadth, with bone exposed and rotting for several inches, were no uncommon sight." If the patient was fortunate enough to have access to sulfanilamide tablets, he could be treated with an ointment of crushed sulfa in oleomargarine. Often the only treatment was amputation.[5]

HE MINISTERED TO HIS FELLOW PRISONERS

held by the Japanese under hopeless conditions while he himself suffered from multiple diseases.

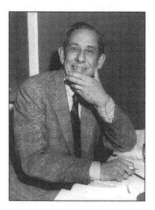

Coenraad F.A. Moorrees. Courtesy Moorrees Family (Louise Berglund).

Coenraad F.A. Moorrees was born October 23, 1916, in The Hague, The Netherlands, the second of two sons and the 11th generation of a Dutch family of patricians that traces its pedigree to the 16th century. His father was a career military officer. As a child, Moorrees displayed talent as a magician, a lifelong interest he passed on to his son. Both he and his future wife, Louise, spent part of their childhood in Jakarta, Dutch East Indies.

Moorrees received his dental degree during the tumultuous years leading up to the Second World War, from the University of Utrecht in 1939. Believing that better opportunities lay in the United States, he and his new bride migrated to the University of Pennsylvania School of Dentistry where, in 1941, he was granted a DDS. Not long afterward, his 2-year internship at the Eastman Dental Dispensary (Rochester, NY) was interrupted by the Japanese attack on Pearl Harbor.

Shortly before Java was taken over by Japanese troops (March 1942), Moorrees enlisted in the Netherlands East Indies Army at the advice of his brother Gustav, stationed in Jakarta as a military physician, who thought that he and Louise would be better off there than being shipped to the front lines. How were they to know that the "front lines" would soon be at their doorstep.

His status as a student did not exempt him from being called by the Dutch government in exile to report to England to assist in the war effort against Germany. To avoid hostile enemy activity in the North Atlantic Ocean, the Moorreeses were sent to the Dutch East Indies via the Panama Canal, the South Pacific, and Australia to Java.

Before the year was up, Dr. Moorrees was imprisoned by the Japanese, and Mrs. Moorrees was interned. As a dentist, Moorrees was allowed to treat his fellow prisoners as best he could, making bandages from bicycle tires. He lived under primitive conditions, he was poorly fed, and he was forced to rely on his ingenuity for survival—all the while saving the lives of others. At one point, he nearly died from bacillary dysentery. He later recalled that tea save his life: ". . . tea, tea, and tea. I survived!"

After the Japanese surrendered in 1945, the Moorreeses were reunited and returned to the United States where

"Connie" enrolled at the Harvard Dental Infirmary to study orthodontics. When he completed his studies in 1947, Moorrees was asked to stay on as acting chief, then, in 1956, he became department chief. Three years later he was also appointed associate professor at the Harvard School of Dental Medicine.

From there, Moorrees found himself involved in an undertaking that charted the course for the rest of his career. Earnest A. Hooton, Harvard University's eminent physical anthropologist, asked him to join an expedition to the Aleutian Islands to study their diminishing indigenous population. The outcome was the prestigious *Aleut Dentition* (Harvard University Press, 1957). His second important book was *The Dentition of the Growing Child*, based on a collection of longitudinal dental casts that were part of a child-health study of 132 subjects from birth to adolescence (Harvard, 1959). His other crucial studies spawned more than 100 original articles, reviews, and book chapters.

Moorrees also established norms for tooth development of permanent teeth based on age and tooth emergence. These data became the standards used by hundreds of investigators studying tooth development. For his contributions to our understanding of facial and dental development—as if to indemnify him for past suffering—he received numerous awards and honors. His most treasured award came in 1985 from Queen Beatrix of the Netherlands, who decorated him Commander in the Order of Orange-Nassau, the highest civilian honor in the country.[6] (There were others who performed thus in captivity, but Moorrees was chosen because of his later achievements.)

HE WAS THE OLDEST SURVIVOR OF THE BATAAN DEATH MARCH

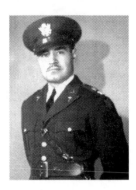

Albert Neir Brown. Courtesy Brown
Family (Margaret L. Daughty).

Albert Neir "Doc" Brown was born October 26, 1905, in North Platte, Nebraska, to parents Albert and Ida Fonda Brown. His mother was aunt to actor Henry Fonda and his father was a railroad engineer. Brown was also the godson of William F. "Buffalo Bill" Cody. He often related the story of sitting on Cody's lap while they shared a bowl of oatmeal.

After his father's death in a locomotive explosion, Brown was raised in Council Bluffs, Iowa, where he joined his high school ROTC. Brown received a bachelor's degree in dentistry from Creighton University in Omaha, Nebraska, in 1927. Brown was drafted into active duty in the military in 1937. He left his wife, Helen, children, and dental practice behind.

Brown and thousands of American and Filipino troops were captured after the Japanese invasion of the Philippines. He survived the Bataan Death March, in which the Japanese forced 78,000 Allied prisoners of war to march 65 miles from Bataan to a POW camp without food, water, or medical attention. An estimated 11,000 prisoners died during the march, including those who were killed when they fell in the jungle. Brown surreptitiously recorded the events he witnessed using a small writing tablet and pencil hidden inside his canvas bag's lining. He witnessed the killing of Filipinos who had attempted to throw fruit to the prisoners on the march. He often wondered how he survived the ordeal while younger men succumbed.[7]

After the Death March, Brown endured a 3-year imprisonment in a Japanese POW camp from 1942 until he was liberated in the middle of September 1945. He was fed nothing but rice while in the lice-ridden camp, causing him to become afflicted with more than 12 diseases, including dengue fever, malaria, and dysentery. He also suffered a broken neck and back. At the time of his release, he was 40 years old and was nearly blind from maltreatment. The once athletic man—he had been a triple letterman in high school—had lost more than 80 pounds, then weighing less than 100 pounds. A doctor told Brown that he would not see his 50th year due to the extent of his injuries.

Brown's saving grace while a POW was his knowledge of radio: He was called on to fix Japanese soldiers' sets. In doing so, he managed to appropriate enough parts to make his own radio, which he used to receive the latest war news from stateside.

After the war, Brown moved to Los Angeles. However, he was unable to return to dentistry or reopen his practice due to the injuries he sustained on the march and at POW camp. Instead, Brown returned to college and began a career purchasing and renting properties. He rented houses and other properties to some of Hollywood's major figures of the time, including Olivia de Havilland and Joan Fontaine. He developed personal friendships with Roy Rogers and John Wayne. He even read for some screen tests while dabbling in acting.

In 1998, he moved from California to southern Illinois, settling in the town of Pinckneyville to live with his daughter. He did not openly discuss his experience on the Death March until the 1990s, 15 to 20 years before his death. In 2007, Brown was recognized as the oldest living survivor of the Bataan Death March by the American Defenders of Bataan and Corregidor, a veterans organization. The American War Library also named Brown as the oldest living World War II veteran at the time. His experience during the march and war was chronicled in the 2011 book, *Heroes of the Pacific War: One Man's True Story*, by Kevin Moore and Don Morrow.

Albert Brown died in a nursing home in Nashville, Illinois, on August 14, 2011, at the age of 105. His wife of 58 years, Helen Johnson Brown, had passed on in 1985. Brown was survived by his daughter, Peggy Doughty; a son, Graham; 12 grandchildren, 28 great grandchildren, and 19 great-great grandchildren.[8] There were eight other dentist survivors of the Bataan Death March, but Brown was singled out here because he lived to be the oldest. This in no way diminishes the contributions and sacrifices made by others not mentioned herein.

HE WAS DECORATED FOR GALLANTRY

for his evacuation efforts under fire at Bataan and Corregidor and for saving fellow POWs aboard a hell ship from drowning.

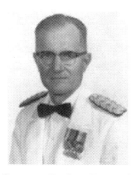

Roy L. Bodine Jr. Courtesy Bodine Family (Regina K. Bodine).

Roy L. Bodine Jr was born in Indianapolis, Indiana, in 1911, the son of a US Army dental officer. He graduated from the University of Iowa College of Dentistry in June 1934. In October of that year, he was commissioned as a first lieutenant in the US Army Reserve. Two years later, he was appointed as a dental officer in the Regular Army. His first duty assignment was the Sternberg Army Hospital in Manila in September 1939. He was captured in April 1942 after the Japanese had overrun the Philippines, being one of 40 dental officers captured. Of the 40, one was killed in Bataan, while Bodine and 38 others became prisoners. Sixteen of the remaining 39 died or were killed in Japan.

Of the 75,000 prisoners taken by the Japanese after the fall of the Philippines, approximately 54,000 Americans and Filipinos made it to their destination, Camp O'Donnell, after a 65-mile trek from the southern end of the Bataan

Peninsula to San Fernando in the scorching heat and having no food or water (later called the "Bataan Death March"). Those falling to the ground in exhaustion who were unable to receive immediate support from their companions were bayoneted or shot. At San Fernando, the survivors were herded into rail cars before walking the last 8 miles.

About 2 months later, Bodine was part of a large group of POWs moved from Camp O'Donnell to Cabanatuan, where about 40 prisoners died every night that first year. Sustained on a diet of rice gruel and sometimes bits of fish, 4 out of every 10 POWs died over the course of the war. His status as a dental surgeon offered no privileges, as he suffered malnutrition, sadistic guards, and the constant threat of illness. Bodine saw his body weight drop from 165 pounds to 86 over the 41 months of captivity.

But the worst was yet to come when the prisoners were loaded aboard ships (aptly named "hell ships") like cattle for transfer to camps in Japan and Korea (See "American POWs in the Pacific," above). Those who survived the merciless conditions were still subject to being bombed or torpedoed by their own countrymen. Describing conditions aboard the *Oryoku Maru*, Bodine wrote, "There were 600 in the large forward hold . . . ventilated only by small openings. . . . They were packed in there without even sitting room, and the suffering without water was indescribable. On the second night, it was a mad house. Many people were crazy, being knocked out by others screaming, knifing, blood sucking; feces and urine everywhere, the sick trampled to death."

Bodine sat helpless in the broiling hold with a friend, John Hudgins, fearing his time was up. "Death was very close and I prayed much," he wrote. "Hadn't confessed for 3 weeks but felt as ready as could be. . . . When bombs were falling and bullets were rattling like hail, I could hear

Hudgins praying at my side, as he repeated over and over, 'Jesus save us.'"

When the *Oryoku Maru* was hit by US carrier pilots, Bodine rescued 16 weakened POWs attempting to swim to shore, for which he received the Bronze Star with *V* (for valor). For his efforts to evacuate the wounded on Bataan under fire, he was awarded the Silver Star. All of these ordeals were carefully recorded by Bodine in shorthand using a Filipino schoolboy's pocket-size notebook and meticulously typed up almost immediately after being freed. This diary was so detailed that it was used as evidence in the postwar war crimes trials.

Bodine was liberated from labor camp at Inchon, Korea, one month after VJ Day and given his choice of stations (he chose Fort Sam Houston, San Antonio, Texas). In 1950, he began research and development in implant dentistry, becoming, in 1958, the sixth president of the American Academy of Implant Dentistry. He retired from the Army in 1961 as a COL after 30 years of service and began a new career as professor of prosthodontics at the University of Puerto Rico. After 10 years there, he spent another 10 years teaching at the University of Southern California School of Dentistry. Now a vigorous 70-year-old, Bodine moved back to San Antonio and took up square dancing and competitive swimming. He outlived all three of his wives. Perhaps his active life and indomitable spirit enabled him to postpone the end until age 94 (May 17, 2005).[9]

Restitution

After the initial euphoria of release from captivity wore off returning prisoners, the question inevitably arose: Should former American POWs be compensated for their slavery and suffering? Or should they simply chalk it up as one of the risks a soldier assumes when he or she becomes a member of the armed forces? At the time, it seemed that the latter was the pill they must swallow, no matter how bitter. As time went on, however, there was a growing feeling that, "by God, the least they can do is apologize!"

British, Australian, and Dutch prisoners held by Japan during World War II have received apologies from Japanese prime ministers and invitations to visit Japan for the sake of healing, education, and understanding. They have also received compensation from their own governments. German companies long ago apologized to those who worked as slave laborers, and additional compensation was paid either by the companies or the German government.[10]

Lester Tenney, commander of the American Defenders of Bataan and Corregidor, wants only the same: an apology and an honorable closure of this dreadful chapter in Japanese-American relations. But since the war ended, the Japanese government has either ignored or denied efforts by American former POWs to obtain either compensation or an apology. Japanese companies have even sought to suppress historical documentation of forced POW labor.[11]

In some ways more troubling, however, is our own government's attitude toward the legal claims that former POWs have filed in American and Japanese courts. In many cases, the State and Justice departments have actually supported arguments by Japanese corporations that the 1951 San Francisco Treaty between the Allies and Japan waived all compensation claims. The State Department has also at times joined with the Japanese Embassy to argue against legislation in Congress asking for compensation from either the American or Japanese governments.[12]

In 2009, a small victory was achieved when the Japanese government issued a formal apology to American POWs and started a "POW Friendship and Remembrance" program a year later, which brings a small group of American ex-POWs and their families to Japan each year to meet with officials and private citizens and, in some cases, visit the sites where POWs were held.

The 1952 Treaty of Peace with Japan provided for modest compensatory payments to former POWs, the money coming from Japanese assets seized in the United States and elsewhere outside Japan. But US and Japanese courts have ruled that the treaty explicitly prevents American POWs from seeking additional damages from either the Japanese government or private citizens.

More than 60 companies used POW labor during the war. Monetary compensation aside, surviving POWs and advocates have been pressing for apologies from more than a dozen of these companies, including some of Japan's largest. But so far, only one— Ishihara Sangyo—a chemical manufacturer, has done so. In 2004 a small number of lawsuits filed in California against Mitsubishi Corp, Nippon Steel, and other companies that used POW labor during the war were dismissed by federal courts.

Survivors contend that Japanese firms like Mitsubishi and NKK have become wealthy industrial giants since the war and should pay for the free wartime labor. For men like New Mexicans Leo Padilla and Cone Munsey, survivors of the Bataan Death March, the situation is particularly galling. Munsey said in a testimony submitted to the House

Administrative Law Subcommittee, "The Mitsubishi company, as an example, for whom I slaved, now owns the copper mines in New Mexico and much, much more."[13]

This is not to say that our government has totally denied any restitution. The War Claims Act of 1948 to adjudicate claims and pay out compensation to American prisoners of war and civilian internees of World War II authorized payments to prisoners of war at the "generous" rate of US$1 to $2.50 per day of imprisonment.[13] No matter how these issues are resolved, no compensation can take the place of those lost years. The least we can do is acknowledge their ordeal.

REFERENCES FOR CHAPTER IX

1   Cimring H. Nor heed the storm. *Cal.* 1962(April);14-17.
2   Nye D. Here's the story of the World War II hero who became the first Navy SEAL. *Business Insider.* (Jul 7, 2015). Retrieved from: https://www.businessinsider.com/heres-the-story-of-the-world-war-ii-hero-who-became-the-first-navy-seal-2015-7.
3   Mauthausen-Gusen concentration camp complex. Available at: https://en.wikipedia.org/wiki/Mauthausen-usen_concentration_camp_complex. Accessed July 18, 2019.
4   In WW2, who treated POWs worse, the Germans or the Japanese? Available at: https://www.quora.com/In-WW2-who-treated-POWs-worse-the-Germans-or-the- Japanese. Accessed March 25, 2019.
5   Bober-Moken IG. American military dentists as prisoners-of-war in the Pacific Theatre during World War II. *Bull Hist Dent.* 1994;42(1):3-12.
6   Ghafari JG. Coenraad F.A. Moorrees: Journey to the top of Mons Scolaris (Mount Scholar). Am J Orthod Dentofacial Orthop 2015;148:210-216.
7   Albert Brown (American veteran). Retrieved from: https://en.wikipedia.org/wiki/Albert_Brown_(American_veteran). Accessed February 20, 2018.
8   Albert Brown (American veteran). Retrieved from: https://en.wikipedia.org/wiki/Albert_Brown_(American_veteran). Accessed August 1, 2019.
9   Roy L. Bodine Jr. (Obituary). San Antonio Express-News (May 26, 2005). Available at: https://www.legacy.com/obituaries/sanantonio/obituary.aspx?n=roy-l-bodine&pid=88855737. Accessed March 11, 2018.
10 Spitzer K. The American POWs Still Waiting for an Apology From Japan 70 Years Later. *Time.* (September 12, 2014). Retrieved from: https://time.com/3334677/pow-world-war-two-usa-japan/. Accessed February 8, 2019.
11 Fifield A. A (very) short history of Japan's war apologies. *The Washington Post.* Available at: https://www.washingtonpost.com/news/worldviews/wp/2015/08/12/a-very-short-history-of-japans-war-apologies/. Accessed August 17, 2019.

12   Treaty of San Francisco. Retrieved from: https://en.wikipedia.org/
     wiki/Treaty_of_San_Francisco. Accessed November 4, 2018.
13   War Claims Act of 1948. Retrieved from: https://en.wikipedia.org/
     wiki/War_Claims_Act_of_1948. Accessed May 15, 2018.

THE SELECTEES—WWII—
POWS—NON-US

HE WORKED AS A SPY FOR MI9

as a Scottish prisoner of war during his time at Colditz Castle, Germany.

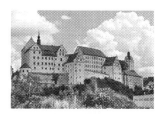

Colditz Castle. Creative Commons.

Born to a Jewish family in Killarney, County Kerry, Ireland, where his father had a dental practice, Julius Morris Green moved to Dunfermline, Scotland, at a young age and studied dentistry at the Dental School of the Royal College of Surgeons of Edinburgh. He moved to Glasgow following his graduation to work as a dentist. Upon the onset of the

Second World War, Green joined the medical unit of the Glaswegian 51st (Highland) Division where he served in the 152nd (Highland) Field Ambulance.

Green's brigade was captured in June 1940 at St. Valéry-en-Caux, France, and he spent months traveling between POW camps providing dental work for fellow prisoners as well as German troops and eventually ended up at Colditz Castle. Shortly after his capture, MI9, a department of the War Office which routinely communicated with POWs, recruited Green as a spy. He would write coded letters to his family and friends in Scotland, which would then be analyzed by MI9 for secret messages informing them of goings-on within the camps. CPT Green proved to be an ideal source to carry out espionage for British intelligence because, as a dentist, he traveled from camp to camp, treating patients and gathering vital information for MI9.[1]

M19

MI9, the British Directorate of Military Intelligence Section 9, was a department of the War Office operating between 1939 and 1945. During World War II, it was tasked with supporting available European resistance networks and making use of them to assist Allied airmen shot down over Europe in returning to Britain. The agents brought false papers, money, and maps to assist the downed airmen.

MI9 manufactured various escape aids that they sent to POW camps. Many of them were based on the ideas of Christopher Hutton, who made compasses that were hidden inside pens or tunic buttons. He used left-hand threads so that, if the Germans discovered them and the searcher tried to screw them open, they would just tighten. He printed maps on silk, so they would not rustle, and disguised them as handkerchiefs, hiding them inside canned goods. For aircrew he designed special boots with hollow heels that contained packets of dried food. A magnetized razor blade would indicate north if placed on water. Some of the spare uniforms that were sent to prisoners could be easily converted into civilian suits. Officer prisoners inside Colditz Castle requested and received a complete floor plan of the castle.

MI9 used the services of former magician Jasper Maskelyne to design hiding places for escape aids including tools hidden in cricket bats and baseball bats, maps concealed in playing cards and actual money in board games. Forged German identity cards, ration coupons, and travel warrants were also smuggled into POW camps by MI9.[2]

Knowing that if he was exposed as a Jew he would be executed, he hid his Judaism by disposing of his identity tags and claiming to be Presbyterian; at one stage, he narrowly escaped punishment for this deception through an assertion from a medical officer that he had been circumcised for medical reasons.

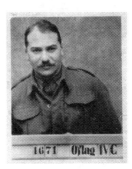

Julius M. Green as Colditz prisoner. Courtesy
Museum of Military Medicine (UK).

His role was to communicate between Colditz and
London through coded letters. Letters he sent to his family
in Dunfermline between 1941 and 1944 would contain lines
that were, to native speakers, effectively nonsense; however,
these were coded messages to be decrypted by Intelligence
staff in London. MI9 provided his family draft letters
to send back to the camp, as well as some from fictional
correspondents invented by the War Office.

German soldiers staffing the POW camps possessed
only a limited knowledge of English, so the code remained
undetected. The letters contained information that was
seemingly innocent—in one, he wrote about a relationship
with made-up girlfriend "Philippa." The language contained
words that, when positioned using a grid system known
as "code 560," would communicate messages to MI9. He
provided information on German troop movements and
railways lines, what troops should bring with them should
they too be captured, as well as which materials should be
sent to Colditz to help POWs escape. He also exposed an
English Nazi informer through his work, who after the war
was prosecuted for treason.

MI9 explained the system to his family in Dunfermline in one letter:

> You will see that in lines 20, 21 and 22 your son refers to certain matters which will have no meaning for you. These remarks are intended for us, so please do not worry about them, nor refer to them in any way when replying to your son. For your private information, we are very glad to tell you that your son is continuing to do most valuable work. Please do not show this letter to anyone outside the immediate family circle and remember to burn our letter when read.

They wrote again in 1944 to assure them Green was "a young man of great resource" and urging them to "try not to worry."

After the war, Green married Anne Miller of Glasgow in 1945 and moved back to Glasgow and worked as a businessman then, later, as a dentist. He wrote a best-selling book about his experiences titled *From Colditz With Code*. Green died in September 1990 at the age of 77.

Spokesperson Julien Roup said that "the risks he was running, as a Jewish prisoner of war in Nazi hands, hardly bear thinking about. Under the surreal humour of his letters lies horror and quite extraordinary bravery."[3]

COLDITZ CASTLE

Oflag iv-c, often referred to by its location at Colditz Castle, overlooking Colditz, Saxony, was one of the most noted

German Army prisoner-of-war camps for captured enemy officers during World War II; *Oflag* is short for *Offizierslager*, meaning "officers camp." This 1000-year-old fortress is in the heart of Hitler's Reich, 400 miles from any frontier not under Nazi control. Its outer walls are 7 feet thick and the cliff on which it was built has a sheer drop of 250 feet to the River Mulde below.

Its purpose was to hold those officers who had proven to be incorrigible at other camps in terms of escape attempts or hostile attitude. Contrary to usual prison procedure, the guards outnumbered the prisoners, and—extraordinary for wartime—the castle was floodlit by night.

In Colditz, the *Wehrmacht* followed the Geneva Convention. Would-be escapees were punished with solitary confinement, instead of being summarily executed. In principle, the security officers recognized that it was the duty of the POWs to try to escape and that their own job was to stop them. Prisoners could even form gentlemen's agreements with the guards, such as not using borrowed tools for escape attempts.

Most of the guard company was composed of World War I veterans and young soldiers not fit for the front. Because Colditz was a high security camp, the Germans organized three and then later four roll calls per day to count the prisoners. If they discovered someone had escaped, they alerted every police and train station within a 25-mile radius, and many local members of the Hitler Youth would help to recapture any escapees.

At first, Colditz was a transit camp for Polish officer-POWs, then for French and Belgians. The first British prisoners arrived in November 1940, and from the outset, they cooperated with the other nationalities in executing a series of brilliant escapes. For example, British LT Airey

Neave and Dutch LT Tony Luteyn disguised themselves as German officers and simply walked out the gate.

Because of the number of Red Cross food parcels, prisoners sometimes ate better than their guards, who had to rely on *Wehrmacht* rations. Prisoners could use their relative luxuries for trade and, for example, exchange their cigarettes for Reichsmarks that they hoped could later be used in their escape attempts.

Oflag IV-C provided the inspiration for both television and movies. This started as early as 1955 with the release of *The Colditz Story*, followed by the TV series *The Birdmen* in 1971, continuing until 2005 with the *Colditz* miniseries. The escape stories of Colditz Castle have inspired several board and video games, such as Escape from Colditz and Commandos. In contrast, the existence of Colditz is virtually unknown in Germany today.[2]

HE WAS DETERMINED THAT THE SPIRIT OF PASSOVER SURVIVE

among his 40 fellow Jewish captives in the Changi prison camp.

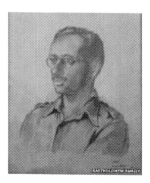

David Arkush. Courtesy Arkush Family (Jonathan Arkush).

David Arkush was the youngest son of Blima and Polish-born Rev Shmuel Arkush, a chazan (cantor) and minister at various UK synagogues. David obtained a dental degree at Liverpool University and, in 1936, began practicing dentistry.

At the outbreak of WWII, he enlisted in the British army, believing that every man would be needed to defeat the Nazis. After basic training, he was posted to Singapore, where he was employed as a hospital dentist and medic.

Arriving at the hospital one morning after being off duty the previous evening, he found that the Japanese had overrun the hospital and murdered many patients and staff. After the British surrender, more than 15,000 Allied troops were imprisoned on the eastern peninsula of Singapore at Changi, an area that had constituted the British military base. Arkush describes the crowded conditions: "Changi consisted of a lot of barrack blocks; they'd been heavily bombed. . . . I don't know how many thousands of men were there, but certainly in the damaged condition there certainly wasn't room for all those men."

He became a POW and was put to work on the infamous Burma railway project, where the captives endured torture and unbelievable cruelty (see next section). Conditions in the hospital were deplorable. According to Arkush, "People who were sick in the hospital, all skin and bone. They were lying on split bamboo—maybe they had a blanket, maybe they didn't. They had dysentery, everybody had dysentery, they lay in their own excreta. Unless they had a pal to look after them, they stood little chance of survival."

In spite of it all, Arkush insisted that Judaism survive. Therefore, he used the knowledge he had gleaned from his chazan father to improvise a seder using sago flour rice cakes, charoset from grated coconut, rice, coffee, maror from mint leaves, hard-boiled eggs, and rice wine.

Every year, he repeated the seder for the 40 Jewish prisoners at the Changi camp in a makeshift synagogue, all the while tending to the dental needs of the officers and men in a dental chair he fabricated out of bamboo. The services continued for the entire 3 years of the railway construction.[4]

By 1945, there were visible signs that the Japanese were retreating. "We heard a noise in the sky and we looked up, and there—you should forgive me—were a dozen bloody great American bombers, flying low over us. . . . This was the first sign our people had seen since we were taken prisoner. And we went mad with hysteria, we shouted and we screamed." For the men imprisoned in the remote jungle, news of the Japanese surrender was staggering and often met with disbelief.

Dr Arkush returned from the war, opened a dental practice in north London, and tried to put the war behind him. But, as his wife, Shirley, relates, "When we were first married David did have nightmares. And he would—like all the other POWs—would not talk about it. And I used to say to him, 'Why don't you talk to me about it? What was it like?' And he would say, 'It was hot.' And I could never get a word out of him."

It was only after they decided to return to Thailand that his nightmares subsided. "We went to the camp about 20 years after we were married. And after that it just poured out of him. . . . I think they feel if they don't speak now it will be lost. David now talks and doesn't have nightmares anymore."

David Arkush died in London on February 4, 2015, at age 100.

Brian Bloom, national chairman of AJEX (the Association of Ex-Servicemen and Women), said that Arkush was "an exceedingly brave and modest man. . . . After the war he actually went back and visited every single Jewish grave he'd buried people in, and said Kaddish over them."[5]

The Burma-Thailand Railway. The Burma-Thailand Railway, also known as the *Death Railway*, was a 258-mile rail line between Ban Pong, Thailand, and Thanbyuzayat, Burma, built by Japan in 1943 to support its forces in the Burma campaign of World War II. Difficult as the undertaking was, it avoided the hazardous maritime route around the Malay Peninsula, where it would be vulnerable to attack by Allied submarines.

Between 180,000 and 250,000 Southeast Asian civilian laborers and about 61,000 Allied POWs were subjected to forced labor during its construction. About 90,000 civilian laborers and more than 12,000 Allied prisoners died.

Because the Japanese had captured many more POWs than expected and did not want to feed and house them, they considered the POWs as an ideal work force for the project. Thus, the railway became the largest single Japanese use of POWs in World War II. Most of the 61,000 Allied prisoners were either British or from the colonies, with only 668 being American. Most of the guards were either misfits, incompetents, or Koreans pressed into duty. Ernest Gordon, dean of the chapel at Princeton University (but at the time a Scottish POW), described the conditions: "The Japanese military violated every civilized code. They murdered prisoners overtly by bayoneting, shooting, drowning, or decapitation. They murdered them covertly by working them beyond endurance, starving them, torturing them, and denying them medical care." It has been said that one worker died for every sleeper (crosstie) laid.[6,7]

DENTAL "IMPROV" IN THE PRISON CAMPS—CABANATUAN

Could dental officers practice their profession while incarcerated? It depended on the camp commander, the availability of equipment and supplies, and the condition of the individual officer. All POWs were required to work, including officers (against the Geneva conventions), so if the dentist, for any reason, was unable to perform his professional duties, then he was assigned other tasks. Those who were permitted to "ply their trade" had to be extremely imaginative to compensate for their lack of instruments and materials.

The former Filipino army training camp at Cabanatuan —at that time the largest POW camp for Americans— offers a fairly typical example.

Initial Setup and Organization. Almost all the dental officers brought into camp some instruments and supplies, which were intended for emergency use. Many had been lost en route, especially during the Death March and in shakedown inspections. On arriving in camp, the officers were required to deposit all these items in a pool, which became the nucleus of the camp dental service. There were no large items such as engines, chairs, or laboratory equipment available. Crude wooden dental chairs were constructed, along with clinic furniture such as shelving. Boxes completed the "reception area." In this manner, the dental service got under way as the camp was being organized, and it was always possible to obtain emergency treatment.[8] Initially, three old, rusty forceps provided by the Japanese were used for extractions.[9]

Treatment of Caries. Since permanent restorative materials were generally unavailable, zinc oxide–eugenol cement (ZOE) was used extensively, with conservation of tooth structure paramount. All this was done with hand instruments. Finally, in August 1942, the first field equipment—a field chair, foot engine, and some supplies, were received. As a quarantine measure, a separate dysentery section was set aside in the hospital for those who were plagued with this disease—including their dentists!

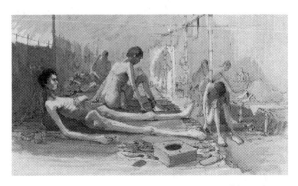

Dysentery hut in Japanese prison camp at Chungkai, Thailand. Courtesy of Tim Mercer.

Dentists as Laborers. Since the Japanese required all the prisoners to work and since facilities and materials were limited, dental officers not occupied at the chair found themselves doing farm labor, putting up fences, repairing buildings, or doing such administrative tasks as sanitary inspections or nursing and feeding the sick. Alfred A. Weinstein, author of *Barbed-Wire Surgeon*, wrote "... Ranking officers, chaplains, doctors and medics were ordered out to sweat and strain under the blazing sun. . . . more and more doctors and dentists gave up their stethoscopes and forceps for a pick and shovel."[9]

Records. Because of the camp paper shortage, dental and medical records were fashioned from 6-ounce American evaporated milk can labels, which had been appropriated in the capture of Manila and were being distributed in limited amounts to the prisoners. After the label was slit and unrolled, its underside, which bore no printing, was used to record clinical procedures.

Alloy. Facing the perpetual shortage of dental alloy, CPT John W. Farley came up with the idea of filing silver coins: Silver was obtained from Filipino coins and other sterling silver objects stashed away by the prisoners. These were filed down with an ordinary file and sifted through gauze. The remaining large pieces were fused and refiled to reduce wastage. A portion (up to 50%) of the remaining large pieces were then added to the supply of commercial alloy.

Mercury—An Essential Ingredient (50%) of Amalgam. One item that was not in short supply was bichloride of mercury. Not needed by the medical department, it was quickly put into use for making amalgam. The mercury was recovered by placing the tablets in 50% hydrochloric acid. A catalytic agent was jury-rigged out of small pieces of mess kit lids. After the whole mass was heated, the free mercury was recovered.

Sterilization. For the first 18 months of imprisonment, native soap and water was the "sterilization" method of choice. The second shipment of Red Cross supplies added an antiseptic to the procedure. No infections from contaminated instruments or unsterilized gauze or cotton were reported. Extractions and other wounds seemed to heal in the normal manner.[7]

Foot Engine Belts. After the supply of foot engine belts became exhausted, a substitute was found in ordinary cotton wrapping string—after trying everything from copper wire to carabao (water buffalo) hide. It had to be fashioned so that it would not twist or knot, jump the pulley track, or unravel. This was accomplished by coating the three-strand, 18-foot endless belt with beeswax, which also made it smooth and strong.

Local Anesthesia. When Manila was evacuated, a large supply of procaine and epinephrine cartridges were taken to Bataan. Even without protection from the tropical heat, at least 50% of the remaining stock was still usable.

Radiography. No x-ray supplies of any kind were received from the Red Cross. Nevertheless, the camp's portable x-ray unit was in workable condition, although exposures could be made only at night when the electric plant was in operation. Without refrigeration, the films were good for only a limited time, with the regular films lasting about a year more than the fast films. Fracture cases, mandibular impactions, and other special cases had priority for the use of the precious 8×10 films, although these were first cut to the size of regular films and wrapped. Owing to fogging, they were of little use for detailed examinations.

Handpieces. The foot engines and handpieces were in a constant need of repair, eventually becoming unserviceable. In the interest of conservation, no mechanical pumicing of teeth was allowed. Fortunately, at least three angle handpieces were received from the "outside."

Burs and Stones. No burs or mounted stones were received from the Red Cross, but a sufficient number of carborundum stones was brought to Bataan from Manila to last throughout the entire period of detention.

Prosthetic Dentistry. Because laboratory equipment and supplies were lacking, no replacement of teeth by bridges or dentures was possible. This created a severe handicap, as many appliances were lost or broken during the campaign.

This only added to the poor physical condition of the prisoners who were thus deprived of the ability to eat.[8]

Oral Hygiene. Only about 10% of the prisoners had tooth brushes. In June 1943, more than 40% of the treatment given hospital POWs was for calculus removal. One dentist kept himself supplied with "dental floss" by painstakingly pulling threads from his clothing.[9]

DENTAL "IMPROV" IN THE PRISON CAMPS—CHANGI

From the remarks of Dr David Arkush: Changi POW Camp, Siam, was established in October 1942. The first prisoners consisted of 1800 men who had been sent from Singapore the previous June with CPT Arkush as dental officer. His equipment consisted of a set of forceps and elevators, a syringe, about six hand instruments, a small amount of local anesthetic, and some ZOE. His dental work was performed out of doors with the patient sitting on a log or a borrowed camp chair.

Shortly after the camp opened, thousands of additional prisoners from Singapore arrived to build the Burma-Siam Railway, so more huts and a hospital were constructed. A special hut was built and partitioned off to be used as an operating theatre, dispensary, laboratory, and dental center. A bamboo dental chair was designed and constructed by a fellow prisoner on the model of the field dental chair with a seat made of rope. The back could be moved forward or backward, and the headrest up or down. A movable bracket table was attached to the chair, and a spittoon was made out of a cut-down 4-gallon gas can. The chair was very strong and was used until the camp closed in June 1945.

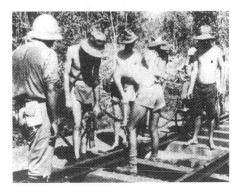

Allied POWs working on the Burma Railway.
Japanese guard at left. Public Domain.

During the 2 ¾ years Changi was in existence, its population varied from a maximum of over 10,000 to a minimum of 1000 men. A large part of the time, Arkush was the only dental officer available. Although the Japanese provided very little, they did supply him with adequate 1 per cent procaine. By administering only about 1 mL of this per extraction, he was able to stretch the supply until other sources of anesthetic appeared. He could, for instance, purchase a few grams of planocaine powder from a small town nearby. He also obtained certain drugs from another dental officer in a nearby camp. Later, the Swiss Consul in Bangkok sent some medical supplies purchased locally. Among these was some percaine which he made up into a 2% solution. Certain supplies such as zinc oxide, some dental needles, and a little dental cement were obtained from underground sources but, in general, he had to use most carefully what he had as he could never be sure of replacing it. Needles were used until they broke. This situation continued until June 1944, when the first consignment of Red Cross drugs from Britain arrived. Included was a large quantity of Novutox, which supplied their local anesthetic needs for some time.

All restorative work was of a temporary nature. Since there was no foot engine, cavity preparation was done with the aid of a right-angle chisel and an excavator, then filled with ZOE. Dentures were repaired initially in Bangkok through an underground source. Later, they were fixed in the camp by drilling holes on either side of the fracture with a broken instrument and lacing the two pieces together with silk floss or silver wire. When this was not possible, the prosthesis was repaired by riveting a piece of aluminum from a mess can over the break. When the plunger of Dr Arkush's syringe wore out, the rubber was replaced by leather washers from the uppers of old boots.

Tooth brushes were scarce, resulting in considerable accumulation of calculus with consequent gingivitis, although very little Vincent's disease (acute necrotizing ulcerative gingivitis) was seen. Apart from a case of cancrum oris in a very debilitated man who died from avitaminosis and malaria, and a fractured mandible caused by a beating from a Korean guard (fortunately, this united without any wiring), Dr Arkush's treatment was limited to extractions, temporary fillings, and gum treatment, although he was once asked to remove a gold crown so that the owner could sell it. He was occasionally asked to treat Japanese patients. When they found out he was unable to make gold shell crowns for their anterior teeth, they came only when in pain.

After 3 ½ years of captivity, he was grateful to be able to return to civilization and to a modern office, with the shortages and improvisations of Changi behind him.[10]

From the remarks of Dr R. I. Mannion: The Japanese made no provision for medical or dental supplies. Such as were obtained, in view of the time constraints, were salvaged from existing British and Australian medical stores and transported on our own initiative to the Changi prison camp. The remainder found its way into enemy hands.

The lack of dental rubber, plaster of Paris, and silver alloy was a serious situation, as many POWs were edentulous, having lost dentures in battle or from the normal wear and tear of prisoner life. Others had their dentition impaired through the loss of many teeth. Fortunately, two resourceful men undertook to remedy the shortages: Staff Sergeant (S/SGT) Masser, a dental technician from Sydney, and a SGT Wentworth who, before the war, was a leading research worker in the Rubber Research Institute in Malaya. Together they produced a silver alloy, a substitute for plaster, and a very serviceable, dark brown dental rubber from the latex tapped from rubber trees growing right within the prison area, red sulfur, and a filler made from filings from a vulcanite rod.

The two "alchemists" produced a substitute for casting plaster from building cement and laterite (a type of reddish clay soil containing iron and aluminum, found especially in tropical areas), mixed with an alkaline solution. The cement was filched from various Japanese construction jobs and smuggled into camp in mess tins, while the alkaline solution was prepared from cookhouse wood ash by dissolving in water and filtering.

For alloy, the three critical metals were silver (obtained from a golf trophy someone had managed to hide from Japanese inspectors), tin (smuggled into camp by captives whose job it was to load Malayan tin ingots for the war effort), and zinc (readily obtained in small amounts from dumps around the camp area). These metals were carefully weighed, smelted into an ingot, and ground into fillings with an emery wheel. Although it lacked edge strength, this alloy proved very serviceable.[11]

VIETNAM—DENTISTRY WITHOUT DENTISTS

What is worse than a POW dentist not having the proper facilities for doing dentistry for his fellow captives? Answer: no dentist at all. When such a situation presented itself in a North Vietnam War prison camp, the prisoners had to rely on self-help dentistry through trial and error, self-experimentation, and a sense of desperation. Sharpened nails, razors, and other homemade instruments were sterilized and used to incise and drain abscesses, relieving acute pain.

One POW sterilized a piece of wire and painfully ran it through his gums to "open dental abscesses." Another got relief by working a fishbone into a painful tooth. Some relief was obtained by placing different kinds of tobacco—such as one might find at the bottom of a pipe bowl—in a cavity. Salt was secretly hoarded to treat infections. Prisoners found that rinsing or massaging with salt water helped relieve the pain associated with dental abscesses. Several men got relief from infected wisdom teeth by lancing the area with a sharpened nail and rinsing with salt water.

The toothpaste issued by the Japanese about every 6 months was often used for more than brushing teeth. It was placed on painful teeth and burns, used as an antacid, to prevent rectal itching from hemorrhoids and pinworms, to clean wounds, and to control the itching and infections associated with insect bites.

Tooth brushes received from the Japanese were of such poor quality that the POWs improvised other tools for their oral hygiene. Charcoal to clean teeth was ground into a paste. Toothpicks were made from pieces of wire, nails, and bamboo strips.[12] Dental floss was produced from threads removed from clothing and blankets.

The above in no way implies that there was a shortage of dental officers assigned to the troops fighting in Vietnam. Of 2817 Army dental officers worldwide, 290 were in Vietnam at any given time. Four dentists and four dental assistants were killed. At the peak of the war, there were 420 Navy dental officers and 790 dental technicians (approximately one-fifth of the Navy Dental Corps) deployed with Marine units. The number of Air Force dentists assigned in Vietnam ranged from 25 a year in 1966 to a high of 53 in 1969 and then back down to 33 in 1971.[13,14,15]

REFERENCES FOR CHAPTER X

1   Julius Green. Retrieved from: https://en.wikipedia.org/wiki/Julius_Green. Accessed January 6, 2019.

2   Oflag IV-C. Retrieved from: https://en.wikipedia.org/wiki/Oflag_IV-C. Accessed February 28, 2019.

3   MI9. Retrieved from: https://en.m.wikipedia.org/wiki/MI9. Accessed January 8, 2019.

4   David Arkush. *pressreader [sic]: The Jewish Chronicle.* (February 27, 1015). Retrieved from: https://www.pressreader.com/. Accessed April 1, 2019.

5   Jackman J. VJ Day anniversary: POW dentist operated with a bamboo chair. *The Jewish Chronicle.* Retrieved from: https://www.thejc.com/news/uk-news/vj-day-anniversary-pow-dentist-operated-with-a-bamboo-chair-1.68135. Updated August 15, 2015. Accessed February 27, 2019.

6   The Burma Railway. Retrieved from: https://en.wikipedia.org/wiki/Burma_Railway. Accessed January 7, 2019.

7   La Forte RS. Burma-Thailand (Death) Railway. In Vance JF. *Encyclopedia of Prisoners of War and Internment.* Santa Barbara, CA: ABC-CLIO; 2000.

8   Fields A. Dentistry at Cabanatuan War Prison No. 1 in the Philippine Islands. *J Am Dent Assoc.*1946;33:1271-1278.

9   Bober-Moken IG. American military dentists as prisoners-of-war in the Pacific Theatre during World War II. *Bull Hist Dent.* 1994;42(1):3-12.

10 Unspoken: the forgotten prisoners of war. Retrieved from: https://mosaicscience.com/story/far-east-prisoners-of-war/. (December 8, 2015). Accessed October 12, 2018.

11 Irons AL. Dentistry in a Japanese prison camp. *Mil Surg.* 1947(Jan);100(1):24-31.

12 Diem CR, Richlin M. Improvisational first aid used by American prisoners of war in Southeast Asia. *J Am Dent Assoc.* 1979;98:535-537.

13 United States Navy Dental Corps. Retrieved from: https://en.wikipedia.org/wiki/United_States_Navy_Dental_Corps#Vietnam_War. Accessed March 30, 2019.

14   The Army Dental Corps in Vietnam. *Dent Stud*. 1967(May); 45(8):720-721.

15   Zimmerman DJ. Air Force Dental Service: A history of high-flying dental care. Retrieved from https://www.defensemedianetwork. com/stories/air-force-dental-service/ Updated May 11, 2015. Accessed December 6, 2018.

THE SELECTEES—WWII—
US—NON-POW

HE GAVE HIS LIFE

to permit evacuation of his aid station on Saipan, killing 98 Japanese attackers and receiving 76 bullet wounds.

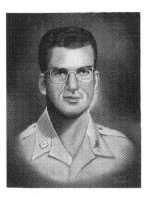

Benjamin L. Salomon. U.S. Army image. Office Of Medical History. AMEDD Regiment

Benjamin Lewis Salomon was born in Milwaukee, Wisconsin, on September 1, 1914. He graduated from

Shorewood High School and attended Marquette University, before transferring to the University of Southern California, where he completed his undergraduate degree. He graduated from the USC Dental School in 1937 and began a dental practice.

He took an interest in firearms: marksmanship, collecting, care, and repair of guns. He unsuccessfully applied for a commission in both the US and Canadian armies. After 3 ½ years of private practice, he was drafted as a private (1940) and served for another year and a half before his commission came through.

In March 1941, still in the infantry, he was assigned to the 102nd Infantry Regiment at Monterey, California. After Pearl Harbor, his unit was transferred to Canton Island, a bleak, barren atoll 1400 miles south of Hawaii, to defend against the Japanese—who never came. To break the monotony of training, training, and more training, commanders organized contests in military proficiency, most of which Salomon won. He was the best rifle shot, the best pistol marksman, the best man with the bayonet, and the best machine gunner in the regiment. He could also strip, clean, and reassemble any weapon in the arsenal faster than anyone else.

In 1942, he was commissioned a first lieutenant in the Army Dental Corps. In August of that year, the 102nd Infantry Regiment's commanding officer declared him the unit's "best all around soldier." In May 1943, he was serving as the regimental dental officer of the 105th Infantry Regiment, 27th Infantry Division, having been transferred from the 102nd. He was promoted to the rank of captain in 1944.

In June 1944, Salomon saw his first combat, going ashore on Saipan with the 105th. As the 2nd Battalion advanced, casualties were high. On July 7, Salomon's aid station was set up only 50 yards behind the forward foxhole line. Fighting was heavy and a major Japanese assault soon overran the perimeter, then the aid station. Salomon was able to kill the enemy that entered the hospital tent and ordered the wounded to be evacuated, while he stayed to cover their withdrawal.

When an Army team returned to the site days later, Salomon's body was found slumped over a machine gun, with the bodies of 98 enemy troops piled up in front of his position. His body had 76 bullet wounds and many bayonet wounds, up to 24 of which may have been received while he was still alive.

Four attempts were made to grant Salomon the Medal of Honor posthumously, but it was not until 2002 that the medal was finally awarded by President George W. Bush. Among the reasons given for declining to approve the award was that Salomon was "in the medical service and wore a Red Cross brassard upon his arm. Under the rules of the Geneva Convention, to which the United States subscribes, no medical officer can bear arms against the enemy." The medal was permanently placed in the Army Medical Department Museum in San Antonio, Texas.[1] The citation:

CAPTAIN BEN L. SALOMON
UNITED STATES ARMY

For conspicuous gallantry and intrepidity at the risk of his life above and beyond the call of duty:

Captain Ben L. Salomon was serving at Saipan, in the Marianas Islands on July 7, 1944, as the Surgeon for the 2nd Battalion, 105th Infantry

Regiment, 27th Infantry Division. The Regiment's 1st and 2nd Battalions were attacked by an overwhelming force estimated between 3000 and 5000 Japanese soldiers. It was one of the largest attacks attempted in the Pacific Theater during World War II. Although both units fought furiously, the enemy soon penetrated the battalion's combined perimeter and inflicted overwhelming casualties. In the first minutes of the attack, approximately 30 wounded soldiers walked, crawled, or were carried into Captain Salomon's aid station, and the small tent soon filled with wounded men. As the perimeter began to be overrun, it became increasingly difficult for Captain Salomon to work on the wounded. He then saw a Japanese soldier bayoneting one of the wounded soldiers lying near the tent. Firing from a squatting position, Captain Salomon quickly killed the enemy soldier. Then, as he turned his attention back to the wounded, two more Japanese soldiers appeared in the front entrance of the tent. As these enemy soldiers were killed, four more crawled under the tent walls. Rushing them, Captain Salomon kicked the knife out of the hand of one, shot another, and bayoneted a third. Captain Salomon butted the fourth enemy soldier in the stomach and a wounded comrade then shot and killed the enemy soldier. Realizing the gravity of the situation, Captain Salomon ordered the wounded to make their way as best they could back to the regimental aid station, while he *attempted to hold off the enemy* until they were clear. Captain Salomon then grabbed a rifle from one of the wounded and rushed out of the tent. After four men were killed while manning a machine gun, Captain Salomon took control of it. When his body was later found, 98 dead enemy soldiers were piled in front of his position. Captain Salomon's extraordinary heroism and devotion to duty are in keeping with the highest traditions of military service and reflect great credit upon himself, his unit, and the United States Army.[2]

HIS DREAM OF ADVENTURE CAME TRUE

when he fought with the Greek resistance behind enemy lines, becoming the most highly decorated dental officer of World War II.

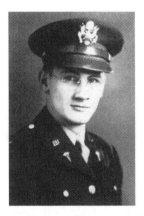

Robert Edison Moyers. Courtesy Dr James A. McNamara Jr, Dept of Orthodontics and Pediatric Dentistry, University of Michigan.

Robert Edison Moyers was born November 12, 1919, in Sidney, Iowa, graduating from high school in 1937. Growing up in central Iowa, Bob idolized the cowboys who came through town with the traveling rodeo. Before entering the University of Iowa, Moyers worked in Iowa City to earn enough money to begin his education. At the age of 17, he enrolled in the honors English program in the College of Liberal Arts. His extracurricular activities included membership in the University Players and serving as student pastor at a small church, earning the nickname "Deacon," a post he continued through dental school.

In the spring of 1943, a few months after graduating from dental school at the University of Iowa, he was called into the military service and assigned to the Office of Strategic Services (OSS; now the CIA). He sailed from San Francisco with his unit via Wellington, New Zealand, and Kandy, Ceylon (now Sri Lanka), to Heliopolis, Egypt. Moyers was not content to finish out the war as a "Cairo Commando." He longed to see combat, having romantic notions about life behind enemy lines. His dreams were about to come true.[3,4]

In late 1943, according to legend, MG William J. "Wild Bill" Donovan was in Cairo en route to the Teheran Conference, when he saw a young dental officer astride two horses in a makeshift rodeo. LT Moyers was quickly recruited into a team needing a medical officer to send into occupied territory in Greece. And the fact that Moyers was good with horses qualified him to traverse the rugged Greek interior where the lack of paved roads required the transport of material for the resistance by horseback and pack animals. His lack of an MD or even postgraduate training didn't seem to faze the OSS.

After training in basic spy tradecraft at the British Special Operations Executive school and the parachute school at Ramat David, Palestine, he was given the code name "Ioway."[4] Moyers thought the date of his first drop was fitting: the second anniversary of the Japanese attack on Pearl Harbor. After several attempts, the four-man team led by MAJ Jerry Wines was dropped into the rugged Pindus Mountains of Evrytania in central Greece. A diverse crew of Cypriots, Russian and Italian POWs, Greek medical students, and two British medical officers soon joined Moyers at mission headquarters in the small town of Domianoi.

Moyers' mission was to provide medical care to the American and British members of the mission and if able, civilians and members of the communist-inspired Greek Resistance movement (ELAS). Despite the loss of medical equipment from faulty air drops, Moyers did his best with what little practical experience he had. His sheer determination to get the job done was not lost on his mission commander, COL Chris Woodhouse. When a British member came down with what sounded like acute appendicitis, Moyers prepared for his "house call" by reading up on how to perform an appendectomy during the 11-hour trip. Fortunately for both doctor and patient, surgery was not needed.[3,4]

During 1944, Moyers' exploits included facing off with Greek resistance leader Aris Velouchiotis, stabilizing a wounded British guerrilla and barely getting him evacuated in time, and organizing building construction teams, all the while suffering from paratyphoid fever, which left him debilitated and, at times, bedridden for days. While in Greece, his observations on the effects of malnutrition on facial growth led him to make it his area of expertise.

After the Germans had withdrawn from Greece, a civil war broke out between the British and ELAS. Because of his good relationship with Greek resistance leaders, Moyers was able to negotiate the exchange of British prisoners and make sure that they were safeguarded during negotiations. For his efforts, he was awarded the Legion of Merit and the

Order of the British Empire. He also received the Bronze Star, Purple Heart, and Order of Phoenix (Greek), making him the most decorated US dental officer of World War II.[3,4]

MAJ Moyers was discharged in September 1945, and he returned to Iowa City to begin his graduate work in orthodontics. He received his graduate degree in 1947 and a doctorate in neuromuscular physiology. He was a pioneer in electromyography at the University of Iowa and was one of the first to track the electrical activity in the masticatory and facial muscles, gaining him the Milo Hellman Research Award and chair of the Department of Orthodontics at the University of Toronto. While at Toronto, he established two research centers. From there he went to the University of Michigan School of Dentistry at Ann Arbor to establish the Department of Orthodontics. In 1966, he founded the Center for Human Growth and Development, an interdisciplinary research center; he served as director until 1980, retiring in 1990. Moyers received the Albert H. Ketcham Award in 1988 and was elected to the Royal College of Surgeons in London in 1995.

On January 8, 1996, Dr Moyers died from a complication of coronary angioplasty. Whether risking his life behind enemy lines in Greece or encouraging his students at Ann Arbor to achieve greater heights, he always gave his utmost.[3,4]

REFERENCES FOR CHAPTER XI

1   Cimring H. Salomon of the Dental Corps. *Tic* (magazine). 1984(Nov);11-12.
2   King JE, Hynson RG. Highlights in the history of U.S. Army Dentistry (2007). Falls Church, VA: Office of the Surgeon General. Retrieved from: http://history.amedd.army.mil/moh/Salomon. html. Accessed September 15, 2018.
3   McNamara JA Jr. Robert Edison Moyers: war hero, motivator, collaborator. *Am J Orthod Dentofac Orthop.* 2015;147:650-652.
4   Clemente JD. Robert E. Moyers: OSS dentist with the Greek Resistance (Code name "Ioway"). *OSS Soc J.* 2010(summer/ fall);34-36.

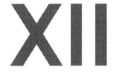

CONCLUSIONS

1. The lack of effective dental care can have a profoundly deleterious effect on the fighting efficiency of troops, yet the US government was a long time in recognizing the need for its troops' oral health.
2. It was also a long time in elevating the status of dental officers on a par with medical officers.
3. One of the few good things to come out of medieval warfare was advances in surgery.
4. Despite their lack of resources, the Confederate dental program was far superior to that of the Union's, largely through the efforts of Jefferson Davis.
5. Historically, dentists have not been properly trained to cope with the demands of military medicine, especially in the treatment of shock, chemical burns, the use of splints, and in administering first aid.
6. The trench warfare of World War I revealed how unprepared military medicine was to deal with the tremendous number and severity of facial wounds requiring specialized treatment.

7. The cruelty exhibited POWs by their Japanese captors during WWII was largely a reaction to the treatment of Japan as a second-rate power by the Western nations following the Russo-Japanese War, their subsequent efforts to restore national pride, and their belief that surrendering was the ultimate disgrace.

8. Dental officers—even untrained troops—have shown remarkable ingenuity in improvising dental "first aid" in captivity.

9. Efforts to obtain compensation for US WWII prisoners' enslavement and suffering have been largely ignored by both the American and Japanese governments.

10. Generally speaking, the Western Powers both dispensed and received the most humane treatment.

11. Thirty-three percent of American prisoners held by the Japanese died in captivity.

12. Putting #11 in perspective, of the Russian prisoners held by the Germans, 57.5% died while in captivity, testifying to the traditional German hatred of the Slavs (notably Russians), whom they considered subhuman.

13. Despite the efforts of humanitarians and lawmakers over thousands of years of warfare, the use of torture to coerce or punish the enemy has not abated.

14. Given the right circumstances, an ordinary person is capable of extraordinary acts.

APPENDIX A

**Selected US Army and Navy Rank
Abbreviations Used in This Book**

<u>Army</u>

<u>Rank</u>	<u>Abbreviation</u>
SGT	Sergeant
2LT	Second Lieutenant
1LT	First Lieutenant
CPT	Captain
MAJ	Major
LTC	Lieutenant Colonel
COL	Colonel
BG	Brigadier General
MG	Major General
LTG	Lieutenant General
GEN	General

Navy

CPO	Chief Petty Officer
ENS	Ensign
LTJG	Lieutenant Junior Grade
LT	Lieutenant
LCDR	Lieutenant Commander
CDR	Commander
CAPT	Captain
RDML	Rear Admiral
VADM	Vice Admiral
ADM	Admiral

APPENDIX B

Notable POWs

Winston Churchill: reporter; captured during Second Boer War (escaped); first lord of the admiralty; prime minister of Great Britain during World War II

James Clavell: prisoner in Singapore; based his novel *King Rat* on his experiences during World War II

Charles de Gaulle: captured at Verdun; POW 1916–1918; French general and political leader; leader of Free French during WWII; president of France

Henri Giraud: French POW of both WWs; escaped German captivity in both wars; WWII general

Rudolf Hess: Deputy Führer of Germany; made bizarre and unauthorized flight to Scotland in 1941, where he was captured; convicted of war crimes

John S. McCain III: American pilot tortured by Vietnamese; held for over 5 years; became a senator; Republican nominee for president in 2008

François Mitterrand: Infantry sergeant captured by Germans in 1940, escaped six times; President of France, 1981 to 1995, longest time in office in French history

Napoleon III: nephew of Napoleon Bonaparte; last French monarch; captured by Prussia in 1870 in Franco-Prussian War

Friedrich Paulus: highest-ranking German general (field marshal) captured in WWII; surrendered Stalingrad to the Soviets in 1943

Donald Pleasence: English film and stage actor. Was shot down while serving as an RAF radio operator during World War II, taken prisoner, and placed in a German POW camp. He later played the part of a blind POW in the film *The Great Escape*.

Jean-Paul Sartre: French writer and existentialist who, as an army meteorologist, was captured by German troops in 1940 and spent 9 months as a prisoner of war

Josip Broz Tito: Austrian soldier in World War I captured by Russians in 1915; partisan leader of WWII; became president of Yugoslavia

Kurt Vonnegut, Jr: American writer captured in the Battle of the Bulge; POW in Germany; one of his novels is based on this experience

Jonathan M. Wainwright: WWII general in command of surrendering Philippine army; captured at Bataan; POW 1942–1945; awarded Medal of Honor; promoted to full general

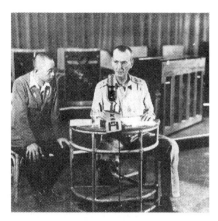

GEN Jonathan Wainwright announcing surrender of Filipino-American forces in the Philippines. Creative Commons.

George Washington: captured in 1754 by the French during the French and Indian War; commanding general of Colonial Army; first US president

Louis Zamperini: Olympic distance runner; crashed at sea during WWII; 47 days on a raft; POW of Japanese for 2 years[1]

REFERENCE FOR APPENDIX B

1   List of prisoners of war. Retrieved from: https://en.wikipedia.org/wiki/List_of_prisoners_of_war. Accessed October 28, 2019.

ABOUT THE AUTHOR

A native of Chicago and a West Point graduate, Norman Wahl was commissioned in the US Army Quartermaster Corps in 1946. After 3 years of service, he worked in the film studios, later producing two documentaries on the history of Los Angeles. He finally decided on a career in dentistry, specializing in orthodontics.

In addition to a BS degree from the military academy, Dr Wahl has a DDS from the University of Illinois College of Dentistry, an MS in orthodontics from Northwestern University, and an MA in history from California State University at Northridge.

He has written for the military and lay presses as well as for dental publications, mostly on orthodontic history. He is the author of *Oral Signs and Symptoms, Wahl's Oral Histories, Who Was Who in Orthodontics With a Selected Bibliography of Orthodontic History*, and articles in the *American Journal of Orthodontics and Dentofacial Orthopedics* (including the 16-chapter series, "Orthodontics in 3 Millennia"), the *Angle Orthodontist*, the *Journal of Clinical Orthodontics, Dental Economics*, and the *Pacific Coast Society of Orthodontists Bulletin*. He has also taught orthodontic history at the UCLA College of Dentistry.

When Dr Wahl heard that fellow dentist CPT Ben Salomon gave his life to permit evacuation of his aid station on Saipan during World War II, he thought, Maybe there were other dental officers who went beyond the call of duty during wartime to prove that dentists were capable of more than filling or extracting teeth. Maybe there was a story here that others should know about. The result was *Dentists at War—12 Who Went Beyond the Call of Duty.*

Dr. Wahl now lives in Provo, Utah, with his children and grandchildren, still busy writing, and editing papers from foreign authors seeking to be published in English-language journals.

INDEX

E

O

P

Printed in the United States
By Bookmasters